I0711080

Welcome to **"The Essential Fertility Cookbook for Couples: Nourishing Recipes to Support Conception and Reproductive Health."** *This cookbook is your comprehensive guide to enhancing fertility and supporting reproductive health through the power of nutrition and delicious, nourishing recipes.*

For couples on the journey to parenthood, nutrition plays a crucial role in optimizing fertility and increasing the chances of conception. This cookbook is designed to empower you with the knowledge and tools to create meals that are not only flavorful but also packed with nutrients known to support reproductive wellness.

From fertility-boosting breakfasts to nutrient-dense lunches, hearty dinners, and satisfying snacks, each recipe is thoughtfully crafted to include ingredients that are rich in vitamins, minerals, antioxidants, and healthy fats—essential components for enhancing fertility and preparing your body for pregnancy.

Whether you're just beginning your fertility journey or seeking to complement medical treatments, this cookbook offers over 150 recipes that cater to various dietary preferences and nutritional needs. Each recipe is designed to be easy to prepare, ensuring that nourishing meals are accessible and enjoyable for both partners.

Beyond recipes, you'll find practical tips on meal planning, ingredient selection, and dietary habits that can positively impact fertility. Our goal is to provide you with a holistic approach to fertility nutrition, empowering you to make informed choices that support your reproductive goals and overall well-being.

Join us as we embark on this journey to nourish your body, support conception, and embrace a lifestyle that promotes fertility and reproductive health. Let this cookbook be your companion in preparing delicious meals that nurture your body and support your dreams of starting or expanding your family.

Warm regards,

Good diet for Fertility essential for couples

A good diet for fertility is essential for couples who are trying to conceive. Here are some key components of a fertility-friendly diet:

1. Balance of Nutrients: Ensure your diet includes a variety of nutrients such as vitamins (especially folate and B vitamins), minerals (like zinc and iron), antioxidants (such as vitamins C and E), and omega-3 fatty acids.

2. Whole Foods: Focus on whole, unprocessed foods such as fruits, vegetables, whole grains, lean proteins, and healthy fats. These foods provide essential nutrients without added sugars and unhealthy fats.

3. Fertility-Boosting Foods:
- Leafy Greens: Spinach, kale, and Swiss chard are rich in folate, which is important for reproductive health.

- Berries: Blueberries, strawberries, and raspberries are packed with antioxidants that can help protect eggs and sperm.

- Fatty Fish: Salmon, sardines, and trout provide omega-3 fatty acids, which support hormone production and improve fertility.

- Legumes: Beans, lentils, and chickpeas are excellent sources of plant-based protein and fiber.

- Nuts and Seeds: Almonds, walnuts, flaxseeds, and chia seeds are rich in healthy fats, protein, and antioxidants.

- Whole Grains: Quinoa, brown rice, and oats provide complex carbohydrates and fiber, promoting stable blood sugar levels and hormonal balance.

4. Healthy Fats: Include sources of healthy fats such as avocados, olive oil, and coconut oil, which support hormone production and reproductive health.

5. Hydration: Drink plenty of water and consider herbal teas and natural fruit-infused waters to stay hydrated.

6. Limit Processed Foods: Minimize consumption of processed foods, sugary snacks, and trans fats, which can negatively impact fertility.

7. Moderate Caffeine and Alcohol: Limit caffeine intake and alcohol consumption, as excessive amounts can interfere with hormone levels and fertility.

8. Supplements: Consider prenatal vitamins or specific supplements recommended by a healthcare provider to ensure adequate intake of essential nutrients like folic acid and vitamin D.

9. Mindful Eating: Practice mindful eating, paying attention to hunger and satiety cues. This can help maintain a healthy weight, which is important for fertility.

10. Consultation with Healthcare Provider: Every individual is different, and dietary needs may vary based on health conditions and other factors. Consult a healthcare provider or registered dietitian for personalized guidance tailored to your specific needs.

By focusing on a diet rich in nutrients, whole foods, and fertility-boosting ingredients, couples can support their reproductive health and increase their chances of conceiving naturally.

Why should couples buy this book?

Couples should consider purchasing **"The Essential Fertility Cookbook for Couples: Nourishing Recipes to Support Conception and Reproductive Health"** for several compelling reasons:

1. *Scientifically-Informed Recipes:* The cookbook offers over 150 recipes crafted with ingredients known to support fertility and reproductive health. Each recipe is designed to provide essential nutrients such as folate, antioxidants, omega-3 fatty acids, and vitamins crucial for conception.

2. *Holistic Approach:* It takes a holistic approach to fertility by integrating nutrition with lifestyle choices that enhance reproductive wellness. The cookbook provides practical guidance on how diet can complement other fertility treatments and lifestyle adjustments.

3. *Variety and Flexibility:* With a diverse range of recipes spanning breakfast, lunch, dinner, and snacks, the cookbook caters to various dietary preferences and needs. Whether vegetarian, gluten-free, or dairy-free, there are options to suit different lifestyles.

4. *Ease of Use:* Recipes are designed to be easy to follow, making it accessible for both seasoned cooks and beginners. Each recipe includes clear instructions and nutritional information, ensuring simplicity and confidence in the kitchen.

5. *Nutritional Support:* Beyond recipes, the cookbook offers nutritional insights and tips on how specific foods can optimize fertility. It empowers couples to make informed food choices that support their reproductive goals.

6. Promotes Wellness: By focusing on nourishing, whole foods and avoiding processed ingredients, the cookbook encourages a healthy eating pattern that supports overall well-being and prepares the body for pregnancy.

7. Comprehensive Guidance: It includes practical advice on meal planning, ingredient selection, and lifestyle habits that can enhance fertility outcomes. This comprehensive approach addresses the nutritional and lifestyle aspects of fertility health.

8. Beautifully Presented: With stunning photography of each dish, the cookbook inspires couples to explore new flavors and enjoy the journey towards conception through delicious meals.

9. Community and Support: Purchasing the cookbook connects couples with a community focused on fertility health. It provides a supportive resource for sharing experiences and gaining encouragement on the path to parenthood.

10. Empowerment: Ultimately, the cookbook empowers couples with the tools and knowledge to take proactive steps towards improving their fertility naturally. It fosters a proactive and positive approach to fertility health through the joy of cooking and sharing nourishing meals together.

By investing in "The Essential Fertility Cookbook for Couples," couples can embark on a journey of nourishment, wellness, and hope, supporting their fertility goals with delicious and nutritious recipes designed for conception and reproductive health.

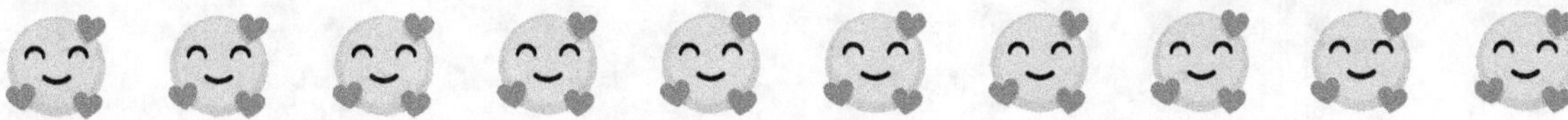

1. Greek yogurt with mixed berries and honey

 Prep Time :   Cook Time :   Servings :

Is this dish easy or difficult for you to make?

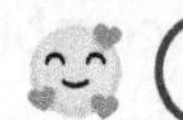 ○   ○

Write 5 friends with whom you want to share this dish

....

....

....

....

....

INGREDIENTS

- 1 cup plain Greek yogurt
- 1/2 cup mixed berries (such as blueberries, raspberries, and blackberries)
- 1 tbsp honey

1. In a serving bowl or glass, layer half of the Greek yogurt.

2. Top the yogurt with half of the mixed berries.

3. Drizzle 1/2 tbsp of honey over the berries.

4. Repeat the layers, ending with the remaining yogurt.

5. Top with the remaining berries and drizzle the last 1/2 tbsp of honey over the top.

This fertility-boosting parfait is packed with nutrients that can help support reproductive health for both men and women:

- Greek yogurt is an excellent source of protein, calcium, and probiotics, which are important for fertility.

- Mixed berries are rich in antioxidants, vitamins, and fiber, which can help improve egg and sperm quality.

- Honey contains natural enzymes, vitamins, and minerals that can help regulate hormones and support fertility.

The combination of the creamy yogurt, sweet and tart berries, and the natural sweetness of honey creates a delicious and nutritious treat that can be enjoyed as a breakfast, snack, or dessert.

Enjoy this fertility-boosting Greek yogurt parfait as part of a balanced diet to help support your fertility journey.

How would you rate this dish?

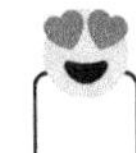 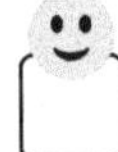 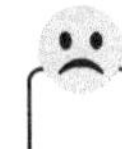 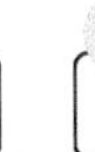 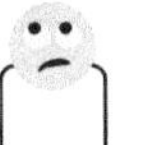 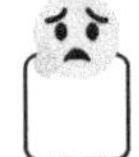

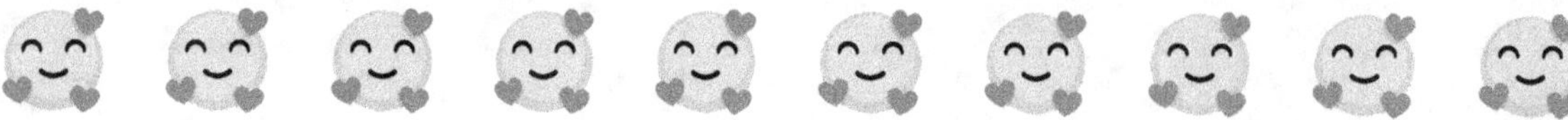

2. Oatmeal with flaxseeds, chia seeds, and banana slices

 Prep Time :   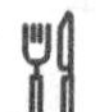 Cook Time :   Servings :

Is this dish easy or difficult for you to make?

◯   ◯

Write 5 friends with whom you want to share this dish

....

....

....

....

....

INGREDIENTS

- 1 cup rolled oats
- 1 cup unsweetened almond milk (or milk of your choice)
- 1 tbsp ground flaxseeds
- 1 tbsp chia seeds
- 1 ripe banana, sliced
- 1 tbsp honey or maple syrup (optional)
- Cinnamon to taste

1. In a medium saucepan, combine the rolled oats and almond milk. Bring to a simmer over medium heat, stirring occasionally, until the oats are cooked and the mixture has thickened, about 5-7 minutes.

2. Remove the oatmeal from heat and stir in the ground flaxseeds and chia seeds. The seeds will help thicken the oatmeal further.

3. Top the oatmeal with the sliced banana and a drizzle of honey or maple syrup, if desired. Sprinkle with cinnamon.

This fertility-boosting oatmeal is packed with nutrients that can help support reproductive health for both men and women:

- Oats are a great source of fiber, complex carbohydrates, and B vitamins, which are important for fertility.

- Flaxseeds are rich in omega-3 fatty acids, lignans, and antioxidants that can help improve sperm quality and ovarian function.

- Chia seeds are high in fiber, protein, and essential minerals like zinc, which are crucial for fertility.

- Bananas are a good source of potassium, vitamin B6, and vitamin C, all of which can help regulate hormones and support fertility.

Enjoy this nourishing and delicious oatmeal as part of a balanced diet to help support your fertility journey.

How would you rate this dish?

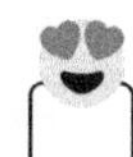 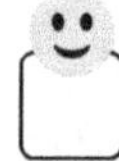  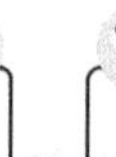 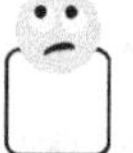 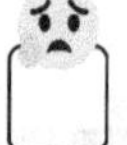

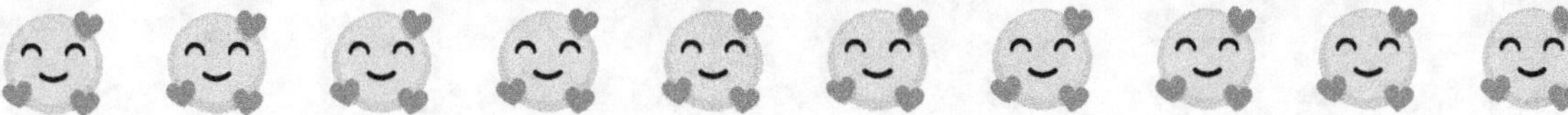

3. Whole-grain toast with avocado and a poached egg

 Prep Time :   Cook Time :   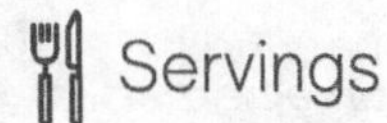 Servings :

Is this dish easy or difficult for you to make?

◯   ◯

Write 5 ....
friends
with   ....
whom
you   ....
want to
share   ....
this
dish   ....

INGREDIENTS

- 2 slices of whole-grain bread
- 1 ripe avocado, mashed
- 2 eggs
- 1 tbsp white vinegar
- Salt and pepper to taste

1. Bring a medium saucepan of water to a gentle simmer. Add the white vinegar to the water.

2. Crack the eggs one at a time into a small bowl, then gently slide them into the simmering water. Poach the eggs for 3-4 minutes, until the whites are set but the yolks are still runny.

3. Remove the poached eggs from the water using a slotted spoon and set aside.

4. Toast the whole-grain bread until lightly golden.

5. Spread the mashed avocado evenly over the toasted bread slices.

6. Top each slice of avocado toast with a poached egg.

7. Season with salt and pepper to taste.

This dish is not only delicious but also packed with nutrients that can help support fertility for couples:

- Whole-grain bread provides complex carbohydrates, fiber, and B vitamins.

- Avocado is rich in healthy fats, folate, and antioxidants like vitamin E, which are important for fertility.

- Eggs are a great source of high-quality protein, vitamins, and minerals like zinc and selenium, which are crucial for reproductive health.

Enjoy this nutritious and satisfying breakfast or snack that can help nourish your body and support your fertility journey.

How would you rate this dish?

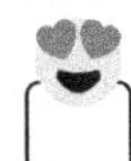 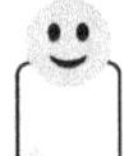 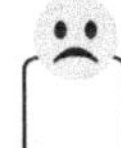 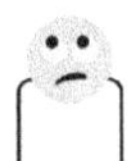 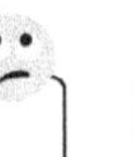 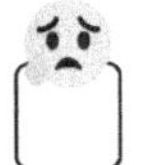

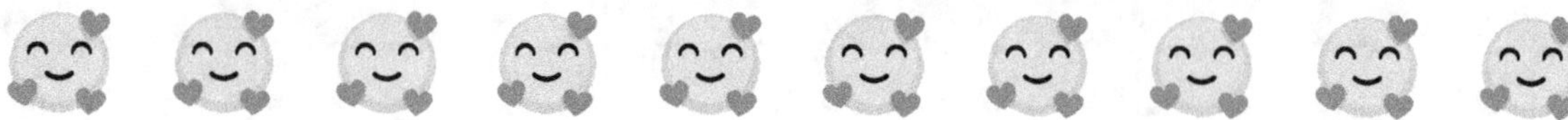

4. Smoothie with spinach, mango, and almond milk

 Prep Time :   Cook Time :   Servings :

Is this dish easy or difficult for you to make?

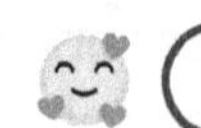 ◯   ◯

Write 5 ....
friends
with   ....
whom
you   ....
want to
share   ....
this
dish   ....

INGREDIENTS

- 1 cup unsweetened almond milk
- 1 cup fresh spinach leaves
- 1 cup frozen mango chunks
- 1 tbsp ground flaxseeds
- 1 tbsp chia seeds
- 1 tsp honey (optional)

1. In a high-speed blender, combine the almond milk, spinach, frozen mango, flaxseeds, and chia seeds.

2. Blend on high speed until the mixture is smooth and creamy, about 1-2 minutes.

3. If desired, add a teaspoon of honey and blend again briefly to incorporate.

This fertility-boosting smoothie is packed with nutrients that can help support reproductive health for both men and women:

- Spinach is rich in folate, iron, and antioxidants, which are important for egg and sperm health.

- Mango is a good source of vitamin C, vitamin E, and carotenoids, which can help improve fertility.

- Almond milk is low in calories and high in healthy fats, vitamin E, and calcium, which are all beneficial for fertility.

- Flaxseeds and chia seeds are excellent sources of omega-3 fatty acids, fiber, and lignans, which can help regulate hormones and improve fertility.

The combination of these nutrient-dense ingredients creates a delicious and nourishing smoothie that can be enjoyed as a breakfast, snack, or pre-workout fuel.

Enjoy this fertility-boosting smoothie as part of a balanced diet to help support your fertility journey.

How would you rate this dish?

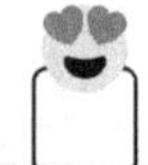 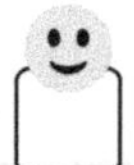 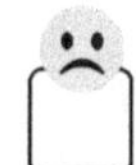 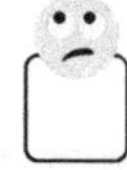 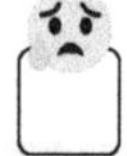

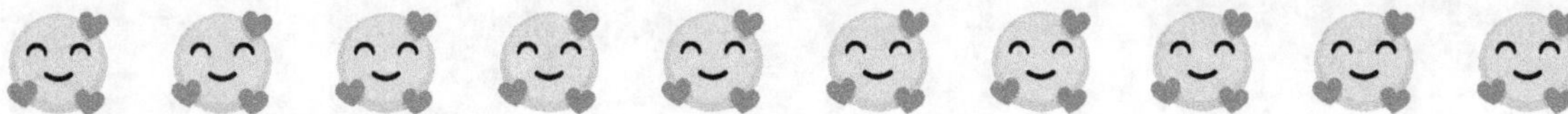

5. Scrambled eggs with tomatoes, spinach, and mushrooms

 Prep Time :    Cook Time :   Servings :

Is this dish easy or difficult for you to make?

◯   ◯

Write 5 friends with whom you want to share this dish ....

INGREDIENTS

- 4 large eggs
- 1 tbsp olive oil
- 1/2 cup diced tomatoes
- 1 cup fresh spinach leaves, chopped
- 1/2 cup sliced mushrooms
- 2 tbsp grated Parmesan cheese (optional)
- Salt and pepper to taste

1. In a small bowl, whisk the eggs together until well combined.

2. Heat the olive oil in a non-stick skillet over medium heat.

3. Add the diced tomatoes, chopped spinach, and sliced mushrooms to the skillet. Sauté for 2-3 minutes, until the vegetables are slightly softened.

4. Pour the whisked eggs into the skillet and use a spatula to gently scramble the eggs, incorporating the vegetables as you go.

5. Continue cooking the scrambled eggs, stirring occasionally, until they are cooked through but still soft, about 3-5 minutes.

6. Remove the skillet from heat and stir in the grated Parmesan cheese, if using. Season the scrambled eggs with salt and pepper to taste.

This fertility-boosting scrambled egg dish is packed with nutrients that can help support reproductive health for both men and women:

- Eggs are a rich source of high-quality protein, vitamins, and minerals like zinc and selenium, which are crucial for fertility.

- Tomatoes are rich in the antioxidant lycopene, which can help improve sperm quality and protect against oxidative stress.

- Spinach is a great source of folate, iron, and antioxidants, which are important for egg and sperm health. Mushrooms contain vitamin D, which can help regulate reproductive hormones and improve fertility.

How would you rate this dish?

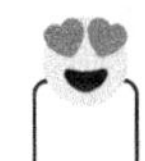 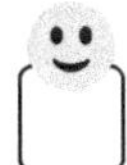 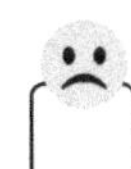  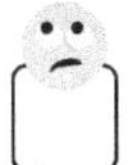 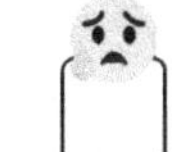

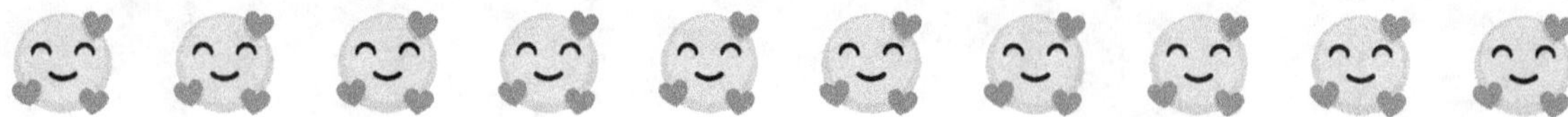

6. Chia seed pudding with coconut milk and strawberries

🕑 Prep Time :   🕐 Cook Time :   🍴 Servings :

Is this dish easy or difficult for you to make?

 ○    ○

Write 5 ....
friends
with   ....
whom
you   ....
want to
share ....
this
dish   ....

INGREDIENTS

- 1/2 cup chia seeds
- 1 cup unsweetened coconut milk
- 1/4 cup maple syrup or honey
- 1 tsp vanilla extract
- 1/4 tsp ground cinnamon
- 1 cup fresh strawberries, sliced

1. In a medium bowl, whisk together the chia seeds, coconut milk, maple syrup/honey, vanilla, and cinnamon until well combined.

2. Cover the bowl and refrigerate for at least 2 hours, or up to 24 hours, stirring occasionally, until the chia seeds have thickened the mixture into a pudding-like consistency.

3. When ready to serve, stir the pudding to redistribute any liquid that may have separated.

4. Divide the chia seed pudding into serving bowls or glasses. Top each serving with sliced fresh strawberries.

5. Serve chilled. The pudding will keep refrigerated for up to 5 days.

Enjoy this healthy, creamy, and delicious chia seed pudding! The coconut milk and strawberries make it a refreshing and flavorful breakfast or snack.

How would you rate this dish?

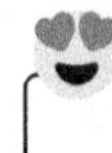 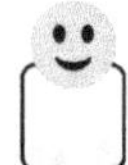 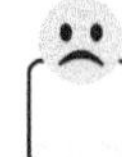 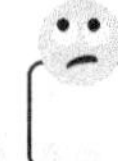 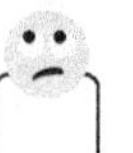 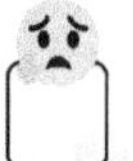

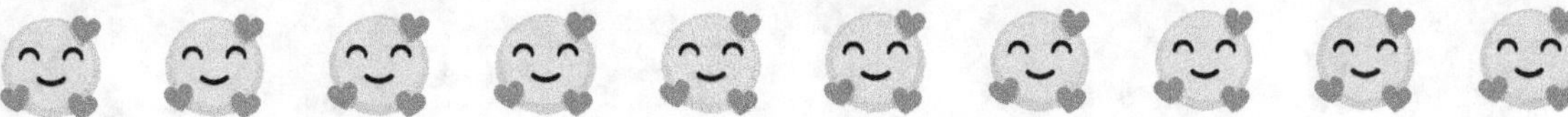

7. Quinoa breakfast bowl with blueberries and walnuts

 Prep Time :   Cook Time :   Servings :

Is this dish easy or difficult for you to make?

Write 5 ....
friends
with ....
whom
you ....
want to
share ....
this
dish ....

INGREDIENTS

- 1 cup cooked quinoa, cooled
- 1/2 cup fresh blueberries
- 2 tbsp chopped walnuts
- 1 tbsp honey
- 1/4 cup unsweetened almond milk
- 1 tsp ground cinnamon

1. In a medium bowl, combine the cooked quinoa, blueberries, and chopped walnuts.

2. Drizzle the honey over the quinoa mixture and gently stir to coat.

3. Pour the almond milk over the top and sprinkle with ground cinnamon.

4. Serve the quinoa breakfast bowl chilled or at room temperature.

This fertility-boosting quinoa breakfast bowl is packed with nutrients that can help support reproductive health for both men and women:

- Quinoa is a complete protein source, providing all the essential amino acids. It's also high in fiber, B vitamins, and minerals like iron and magnesium, which are important for fertility.

- Blueberries are rich in antioxidants, vitamins, and fiber, which can help improve egg and sperm quality.

- Walnuts are a great source of omega-3 fatty acids, which can help regulate hormones and improve fertility.

- Cinnamon has anti-inflammatory properties and can help regulate blood sugar levels, which is important for fertility.

- Honey contains natural enzymes, vitamins, and minerals that can help support overall reproductive health.

Enjoy this nourishing and delicious quinoa breakfast bowl as part of a balanced diet to help support your fertility journey.

How would you rate this dish?

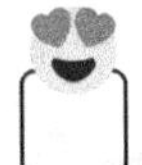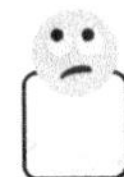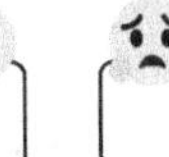

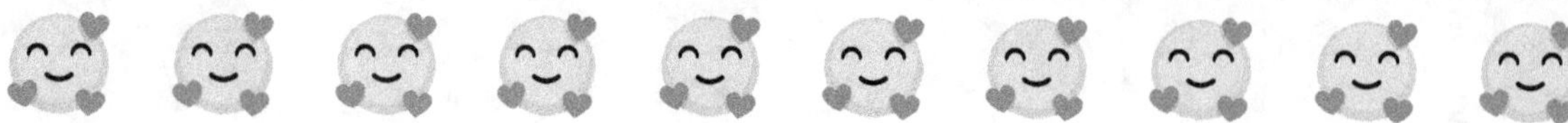

8. Cottage cheese with pineapple chunks and a drizzle of honey

 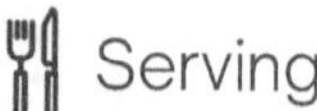 Prep Time :   Cook Time :   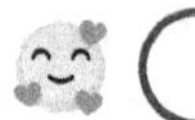 Servings :

Is this dish easy or difficult for you to make?

 ◯   ◯

Write 5 friends with whom you want to share this dish

....

....

....

....

....

INGREDIENTS

- 1 cup low-fat cottage cheese
- 1/2 cup fresh pineapple chunks
- 1 tbsp honey

1. In a small bowl, scoop the cottage cheese and top with the fresh pineapple chunks.

2. Drizzle the honey over the top of the cottage cheese and pineapple.

This simple and delicious dish is packed with nutrients that can help support fertility for couples:

- Cottage cheese is an excellent source of protein, calcium, and vitamin B12, all of which are important for reproductive health.

- Pineapple is rich in the enzyme bromelain, which can help reduce inflammation and improve fertility in both men and women.

- Honey contains natural antioxidants, vitamins, and minerals that can help regulate hormones and support overall fertility.

The combination of the creamy cottage cheese, sweet pineapple, and the natural sweetness of honey creates a nourishing and satisfying snack or light meal.

Enjoy this fertility-boosting cottage cheese dish as part of a balanced diet to help support your fertility journey. The simplicity of the recipe makes it an easy and convenient option to incorporate into your daily routine.

How would you rate this dish?

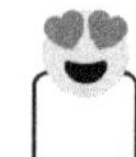 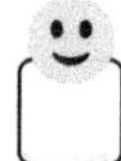 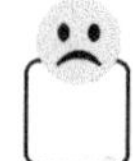 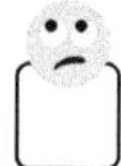 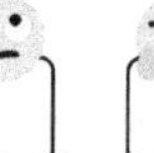 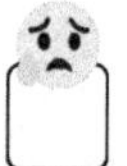

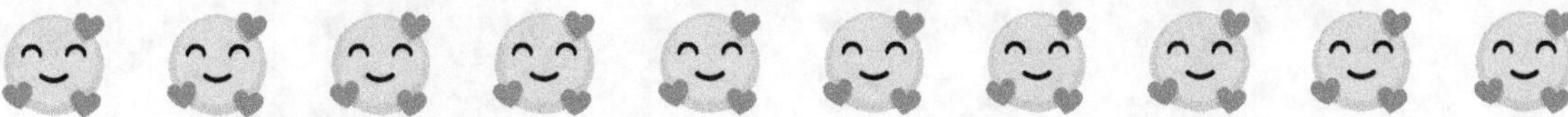

9. Whole-grain pancakes with fresh raspberries

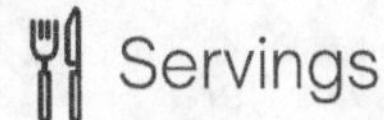 Prep Time :   Cook Time :   Servings :

Is this dish easy or difficult for you to make?

 ○   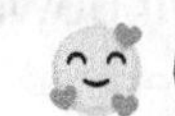 ○

Write 5
friends
with
whom
you
want to
share
this
dish

INGREDIENTS

- 1 cup whole-wheat flour
- 1 tsp baking powder
- 1/4 tsp baking soda
- 1/4 tsp salt
- 1 egg
- 1 cup unsweetened almond milk
- 1 tbsp honey
- 1 tsp vanilla extract
- 1 cup fresh raspberries

1. In a medium bowl, whisk together the whole-wheat flour, baking powder, baking soda, and salt.

2. In a separate bowl, beat the egg. Then stir in the almond milk, honey, and vanilla extract.

3. Pour the wet ingredients into the dry ingredients and mix just until combined (do not overmix).

4. Heat a lightly oiled non-stick skillet or griddle over medium heat.

5. Scoop about 1/4 cup of the batter onto the hot surface and cook for 2-3 minutes, or until bubbles start to form on the surface.

6. Flip the pancake and cook for an additional 1-2 minutes, until golden brown.

7. Repeat with the remaining batter, making about 8-10 pancakes total.

8. Serve the whole-grain pancakes warm, topped with fresh raspberries.

This fertility-boosting pancake dish is packed with nutrients that can help support reproductive health for both men and women:

- Whole-wheat flour is high in fiber, B vitamins, and mInerals like zinc, which are important for fertility.
- Raspberries are rich in antioxidants, vitamins, and fiber, which can help improve egg and sperm quality.
- Honey contains natural enzymes, vitamins, and minerals that can help regulate hormones and support fertility.
- Almond milk is low in calories and high in healthy fats, vitamin E, and calcium, which are all beneficial for fertility.

How would you rate this dish?

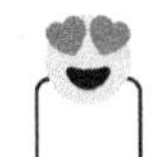 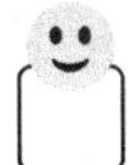  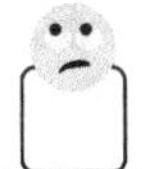 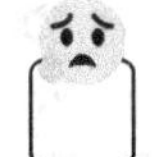

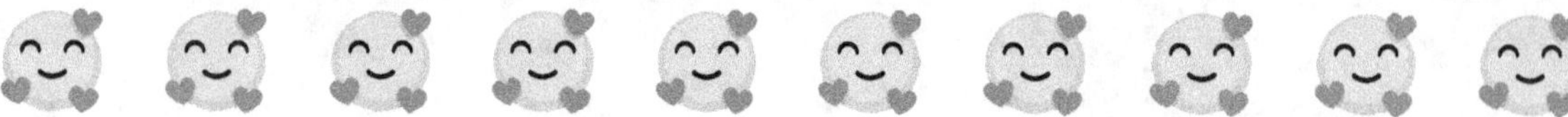

10. Spinach and feta omelet with whole-grain toast

 Prep Time :    Cook Time :   Servings :

Is this dish easy or difficult for you to make?

Write 5 friends with whom you want to share this dish

....

....

....

....

INGREDIENTS

- 3 large eggs
- 1 tbsp olive oil
- 1 cup fresh spinach leaves, chopped
- 2 tbsp crumbled feta cheese
- 2 slices of whole-grain bread, toasted

How would you rate this dish?

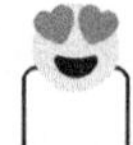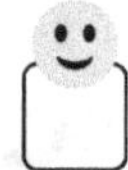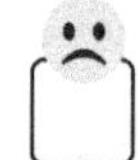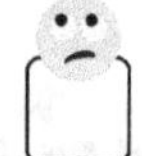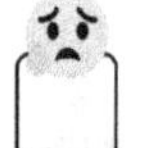

1. Crack the eggs into a small bowl and beat them lightly with a fork until well combined.

2. Heat the olive oil in a non-stick skillet over medium heat.

3. Pour the beaten eggs into the skillet and let them sit for 30 seconds to a minute, until the edges start to set.

4. Using a spatula, gently push the cooked egg towards the center of the skillet, tilting the pan to allow the uncooked egg to flow to the edges.

5. Once the eggs are mostly set but still a bit runny on top, sprinkle the chopped spinach and crumbled feta cheese over the top.

6. Fold the omelet in half and slide it onto a plate. Serve the spinach and feta omelet with the toasted whole-grain bread.

This fertility-boosting omelet dish is packed with nutrients that can help support reproductive health for both men and women:

- Eggs are a rich source of high-quality protein, vitamins, and minerals like zinc and selenium, which are crucial for fertility.
- Spinach is a great source of folate, iron, and antioxidants, which are important for egg and sperm health.
- Feta cheese is a good source of protein, calcium, and vitamin B12, all of which can help improve fertility.
- Whole-grain toast provides complex carbohydrates, fiber, and B vitamins, which are important for overall reproductive function.

Enjoy this delicious and nutritious spinach and feta omelet with whole-grain toast as part of a balanced diet to help support your fertility journey.

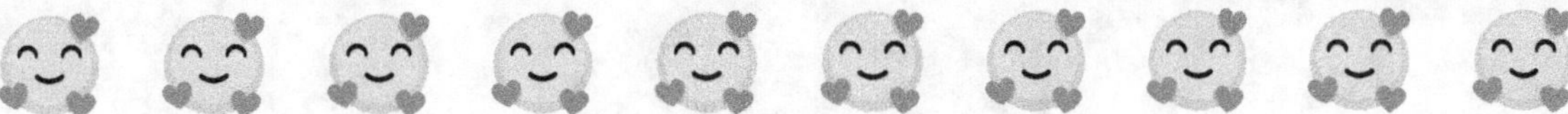

11. Quinoa salad with chickpeas, cucumber, and feta

 *Let's do that and fill in the time here* Prep Time :   Cook Time: 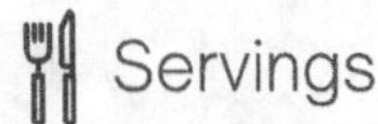 Servings :

Is this dish easy or difficult for you to make?

○   ○

Write 5 friends with whom you want to share this dish

....

....

....

....

....

INGREDIENTS

- 1 cup cooked quinoa, cooled
- 1 (15 oz) can chickpeas, rinsed and drained
- 1 cup diced cucumber
- 1/4 cup crumbled feta cheese
- 2 tbsp chopped fresh parsley
- 2 tbsp olive oil
- 1 tbsp lemon juice
- 1 tsp Dijon mustard
- Salt and pepper to taste

How would you rate this dish?

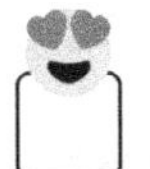   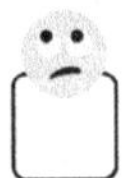 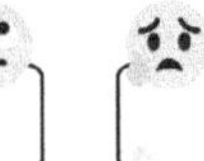 

1. In a large bowl, combine the cooked quinoa, chickpeas, diced cucumber, crumbled feta, and chopped parsley.

2. In a small bowl, whisk together the olive oil, lemon juice, and Dijon mustard. Season with salt and pepper to taste.

3. Pour the dressing over the quinoa salad and toss gently to coat.

4. Refrigerate the salad for at least 30 minutes to allow the flavors to meld.

5. Serve chilled or at room temperature.

This fertility-boosting quinoa salad is packed with nutrients that can help support reproductive health for both men and women:

- Quinoa is a complete protein source, providing all the essential amino acids. It's also high in fiber, B vitamins, and minerals like iron and magnesium, which are important for fertility.

- Chickpeas are a good source of protein, fiber, and folate, which can help improve egg and sperm quality.

- Cucumber is rich in water, vitamins, and antioxidants, which can help reduce inflammation and support overall reproductive function.

- Feta cheese is a good source of protein, calcium, and vitamin B12, all of which can help improve fertility.

- Olive oil and lemon juice provide healthy fats and vitamin C, respectively, which are important for hormone regulation and fertility.

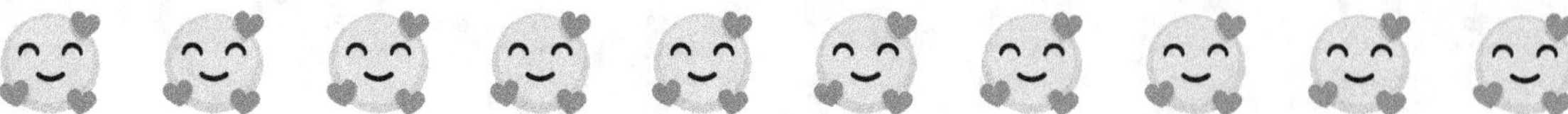

12. Lentil soup with carrots, celery, and onions

Let's do that and fill in the time here  Prep Time :  Cook Time : Servings :

Is this dish easy or difficult for you to make?

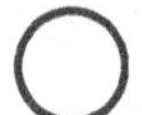 ◯ 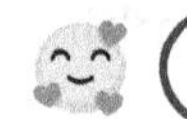 ◯

Write 5 friends with whom you want to share this dish
....
....
....
....
....

INGREDIENTS

- 1 cup dry brown or green lentils, rinsed
- 4 cups low-sodium vegetable broth
- 1 tbsp olive oil
- 1 onion, diced
- 2 carrots, peeled and diced
- 2 celery stalks, diced
- 3 garlic cloves, minced
- 1 tsp ground cumin
- 1 tsp dried thyme
- Salt and pepper to taste
- Chopped parsley for garnish (optional)

How would you rate this dish?

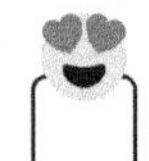 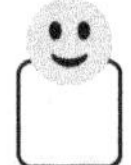 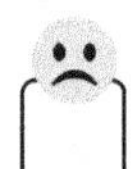 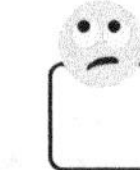 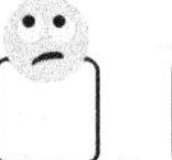 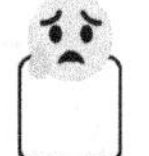

1. In a large pot, bring the vegetable broth to a boil over high heat. Add the rinsed lentils, reduce heat to medium-low, and simmer for 20-25 minutes, or until the lentils are tender.

2. In a separate skillet, heat the olive oil over medium heat. Add the diced onion, carrots, and celery. Sauté for 5-7 minutes, until the vegetables are softened.

3. Add the minced garlic to the vegetable mixture and cook for an additional minute, until fragrant.

4. Transfer the sautéed vegetables to the pot with the cooked lentils. Stir in the ground cumin and dried thyme.

5. Season the soup with salt and pepper to taste.

6. Simmer the lentil soup for an additional 10 minutes to allow the flavors to meld.

7. Serve the lentil soup hot, garnished with chopped parsley if desired.

This fertility-boosting lentil soup is packed with nutrients that can help support reproductive health for both men and women:

- Lentils are a great source of protein, fiber, folate, and iron, all of which are important for fertility.
- Carrots are rich in beta-carotene, which can help improve egg and sperm quality.
- Celery is a good source of antioxidants and vitamins that can help regulate hormones and reduce inflammation.
- Onions and garlic contain sulfur-containing compounds that can help improve sperm motility and quality.
- Cumin and thyme are both herbs that have been shown to have fertility-enhancing properties.

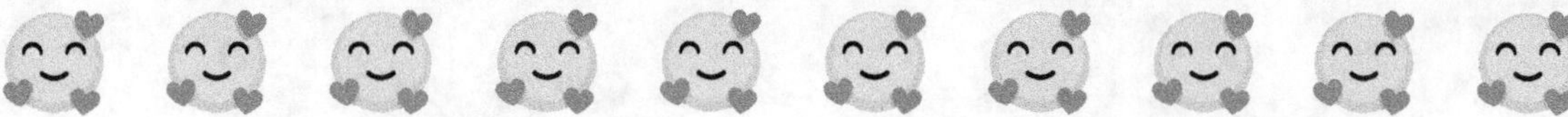

13. Grilled chicken salad with mixed greens and avocado

 Prep Time :    Cook Time :   Servings :

Is this dish easy or difficult for you to make?

⭘   ⭘

Write 5 friends with whom you want to share this dish
....
....
....
....
....

INGREDIENTS

- 4 boneless, skinless chicken breasts
- 1 tbsp olive oil
- 1 tsp dried oregano
- Salt and pepper to taste
- 6 cups mixed greens (such as spinach, arugula, and kale)
- 1 avocado, sliced
- 1/4 cup crumbled feta cheese
- 2 tbsp balsamic vinaigrette

1. Preheat your grill or grill pan to medium-high heat.

2. Brush the chicken breasts with olive oil and season them with dried oregano, salt, and pepper.

3. Grill the chicken for 5-7 minutes per side, or until it's cooked through and reaches an internal temperature of 165°F.

4. Remove the chicken from the grill and let it rest for a few minutes before slicing it into strips.

5. In a large salad bowl, combine the mixed greens, sliced avocado, and crumbled feta cheese.

6. Top the salad with the grilled chicken strips.

7. Drizzle the balsamic vinaigrette over the top of the salad and toss gently to coat.

This fertility-boosting grilled chicken salad is packed with nutrients that can help support reproductive health for both men and women:

- Chicken is a lean protein source that can help support overall fertility.
- Mixed greens, such as spinach and kale, are rich in folate, iron, and antioxidants, which are important for egg and sperm health.
- Avocado is a great source of healthy fats, vitamins, and minerals that can help regulate hormones and improve fertility.
- Feta cheese is a good source of protein, calcium, and vitamin B12, all of which can help improve fertility.
- Balsamic vinegar contains polyphenols that can help reduce inflammation and support overall reproductive function.

How would you rate this dish?

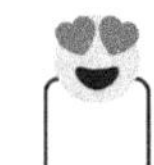 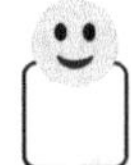 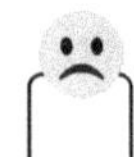 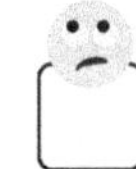 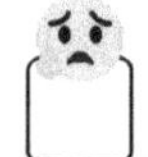

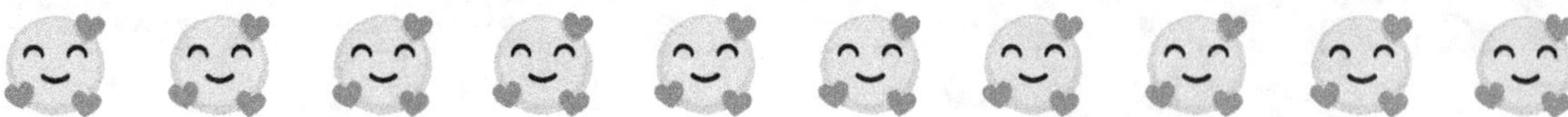

14. Tuna salad with mixed greens and olive oil dressing

 Prep Time :   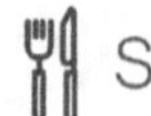 Cook Time :   Servings :

Is this dish easy or difficult for you to make?

Write 5 friends with whom you want to share this dish ....

INGREDIENTS

- 1 (5 oz) can of tuna, drained and flaked
- 2 tbsp olive oil
- 1 tbsp lemon juice
- 1 tsp Dijon mustard
- 1 tbsp chopped fresh parsley
- Salt and pepper to taste
- 4 cups mixed greens (such as spinach, arugula, and kale)
- 1/4 cup sliced cucumber
- 2 tbsp crumbled feta cheese

Dressing:
- 2 tbsp olive oil
- 1 tbsp balsamic vinegar
- 1 tsp honey
- Salt and pepper to taste

How would you rate this dish?

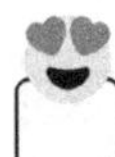 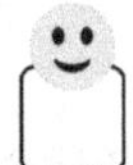 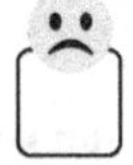 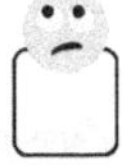 

1. In a medium bowl, combine the flaked tuna, 2 tbsp olive oil, lemon juice, Dijon mustard, and chopped parsley. Season with salt and pepper to taste.

2. In a large salad bowl, arrange the mixed greens, sliced cucumber, and crumbled feta cheese.

3. In a small bowl, whisk together the ingredients for the dressing: 2 tbsp olive oil, balsamic vinegar, honey, and salt and pepper.

4. Drizzle the dressing over the salad and toss gently to coat. Top the salad with the tuna mixture.

This fertility-boosting tuna salad is packed with nutrients that can help support reproductive health for both men and women:

- Tuna is a great source of high-quality protein, omega-3 fatty acids, and selenium, which are all important for fertility.

- Mixed greens, such as spinach and arugula, are rich in folate, iron, and antioxidants, which can help improve egg and sperm quality.

- Cucumber is hydrating and contains vitamins and minerals that can help reduce inflammation and support overall reproductive function.

- Feta cheese is a good source of protein, calcium, and vitamin B12, all of which can help improve fertility.

- Olive oil and balsamic vinegar provide healthy fats and antioxidants that can help regulate hormones and support fertility.

Enjoy this delicious and nutritious tuna salad as part of a balanced diet to help support your fertility journey.

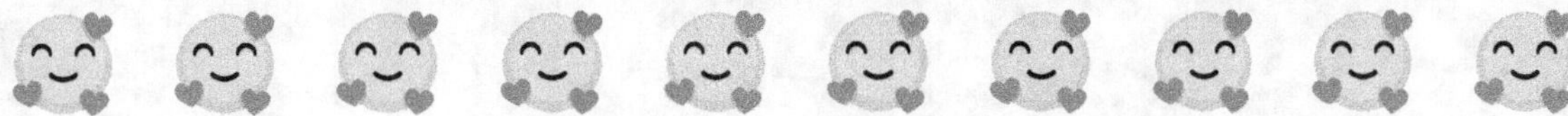

15. Spinach and strawberry salad with walnuts and balsamic vinaigrette

Let's do that and fill in the time here  Prep Time :    Cook Time :   Servings :

Is this dish easy or difficult for you to make?

Write 5 friends with whom you want to share this dish

....
....
....
....
....

INGREDIENTS

- 5 cups fresh spinach leaves
- 1 cup fresh strawberries, sliced
- 1/4 cup chopped walnuts
- 2 tbsp crumbled feta cheese
- Balsamic Vinaigrette:
- 2 tbsp balsamic vinegar
- 1 tbsp olive oil
- 1 tsp Dijon mustard
- 1 tsp honey
- Salt and pepper to taste

How would you rate this dish?

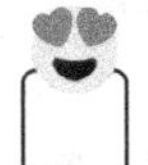 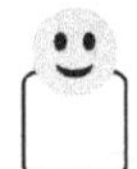  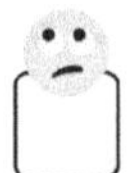 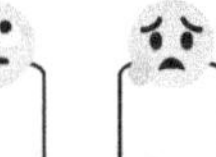

1. In a large salad bowl, combine the fresh spinach leaves, sliced strawberries, chopped walnuts, and crumbled feta cheese.

2. In a small bowl, whisk together the ingredients for the balsamic vinaigrette: balsamic vinegar, olive oil, Dijon mustard, honey, and salt and pepper to taste.

3. Drizzle the balsamic vinaigrette over the salad and toss gently to coat.

This fertility-boosting spinach and strawberry salad is packed with nutrients that can help support reproductive health for both men and women:

- Spinach is a rich source of folate, iron, and antioxidants, which are important for egg and sperm health.

- Strawberries are high in vitamin C, an antioxidant that can help improve sperm quality and protect against oxidative stress.

- Walnuts are a great source of omega-3 fatty acids, which can help regulate hormones and improve fertility.

- Feta cheese is a good source of protein, calcium, and vitamin B12, all of which can help improve fertility.

- Balsamic vinegar contains polyphenols that can help reduce inflammation and support overall reproductive function.

- Olive oil and honey provide healthy fats and natural sweetness that can help balance hormones and support fertility.

Enjoy this delicious and nutritious spinach and strawberry salad as part of a balanced diet to help support your fertility journey.

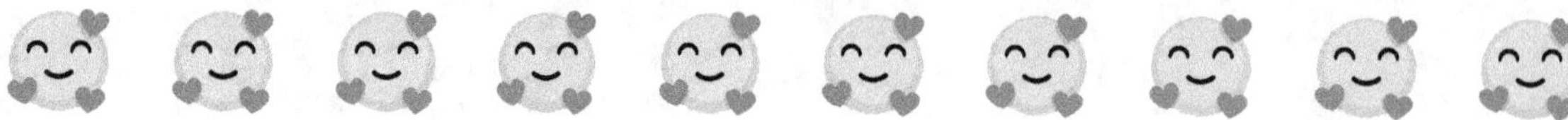

16. Turkey and avocado wrap with whole-grain tortilla

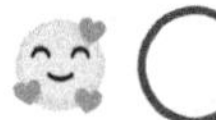 Prep Time :   Cook Time :   Servings :

Is this dish easy or difficult for you to make?

 ○   ⊙ ○

Write 5 ....
friends
with ....
whom
you ....
want to
share ....
this
dish ....

INGREDIENTS

- 1 whole-grain tortilla or wrap
- 2-3 slices of turkey breast
- 1/2 avocado, sliced
- 1 tbsp hummus
- 1/4 cup baby spinach leaves
- 1 tbsp crumbled feta cheese
- Salt and pepper to taste

How would you rate this dish?

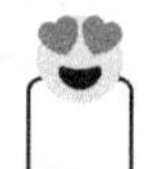 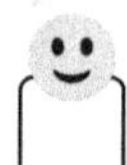 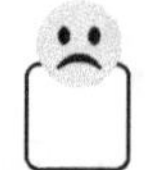 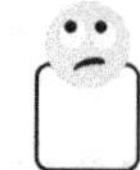 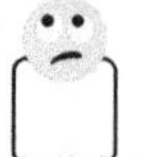 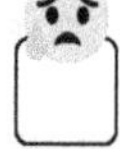

1. Lay the whole-grain tortilla or wrap on a flat surface.

2. Spread the hummus evenly over the center of the tortilla.

3. Layer the turkey slices, avocado slices, baby spinach leaves, and crumbled feta cheese on top of the hummus.

4. Season with salt and pepper to taste.

5. Fold the bottom of the tortilla up over the filling, then fold in the sides and continue rolling tightly to create a wrap.

This fertility-boosting turkey and avocado wrap is packed with nutrients that can help support reproductive health for both men and women:

- Whole-grain tortilla provides complex carbohydrates, fiber, and B vitamins, which are important for fertility.

- Turkey is a lean protein source that can help support overall reproductive function.

- Avocado is rich in healthy fats, vitamins, and minerals that can help regulate hormones and improve fertility.

- Spinach is a great source of folate, iron, and antioxidants, which are important for egg and sperm health.

- Feta cheese is a good source of protein, calcium, and vitamin B12, all of which can help improve fertility.

- Hummus is a nutritious spread that provides protein, fiber, and healthy fats to support fertility.

Enjoy this delicious and nourishing turkey and avocado wrap as part of a balanced diet to help support your fertility journey.

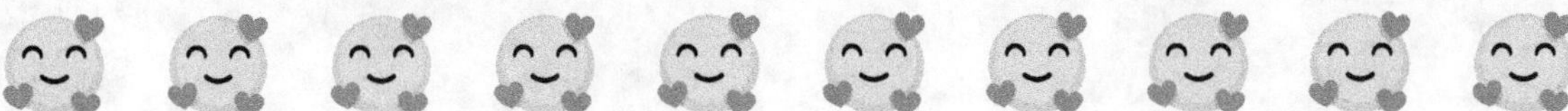

17. Black bean and corn salad with lime dressing

🕐 Prep Time : 🕐 Cook Time : 🍴 Servings :

Is this dish easy or difficult for you to make?

 ⭕   😊 ⭕

Write 5 friends with whom you want to share this dish

....
....
....
....
....

INGREDIENTS

- 1 (15 oz) can black beans, rinsed and drained
- 1 cup frozen corn, thawed
- 1 red bell pepper, diced
- 1/2 red onion, diced
- 1/4 cup chopped fresh cilantro
- Dressing:
- 2 tbsp olive oil
- 2 tbsp lime juice
- 1 tsp Dijon mustard
- 1 tsp honey
- Salt and pepper to taste

How would you rate this dish?

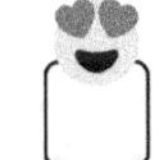 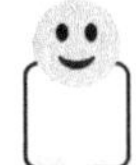 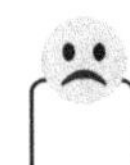 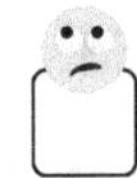 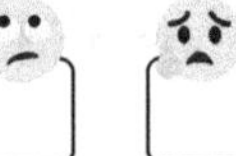

1. In a large bowl, combine the rinsed and drained black beans, thawed corn, diced red bell pepper, diced red onion, and chopped fresh cilantro.

2. In a small bowl, whisk together the ingredients for the dressing: olive oil, lime juice, Dijon mustard, honey, and salt and pepper to taste.

3. Pour the dressing over the black bean and corn salad and toss gently to coat.

4. Refrigerate the salad for at least 30 minutes to allow the flavors to meld. Serve chilled or at room temperature.

This fertility-boosting black bean and corn salad is packed with nutrients that can help support reproductive health for both men and women:

- Black beans are a great source of protein, fiber, and folate, which are important for fertility.

- Corn is rich in antioxidants, vitamins, and minerals that can help improve egg and sperm quality.

- Red bell pepper is a good source of vitamin C, an antioxidant that can help protect against oxidative stress and support fertility.

- Red onion contains sulfur-containing compounds that can help improve sperm motility and quality.

- Cilantro is an herb that has been shown to have anti-inflammatory properties and can help regulate hormones.

- Olive oil and lime juice provide healthy fats and vitamin C, respectively, which are important for hormone regulation and fertility.

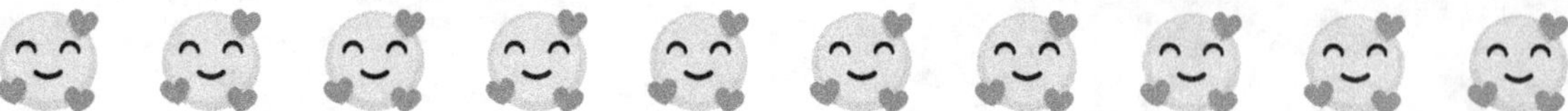

18. Grilled salmon salad with arugula and quinoa

Prep Time :   Cook Time :   Servings :

Is this dish easy or difficult for you to make?

 ○    ○

Write 5 ....
friends
with ....
whom
you ....
want to
share ....
this
dish ....

INGREDIENTS

- 4 oz grilled salmon fillet
- 2 cups baby arugula
- 1/2 cup cooked quinoa
- 1/4 cup sliced cucumber
- 2 tbsp crumbled feta cheese
- 1 tbsp chopped walnuts
- Dressing:
- 1 tbsp olive oil
- 1 tbsp balsamic vinegar
- 1 tsp Dijon mustard
- 1 tsp honey
- Salt and pepper to taste

How would you rate this dish?

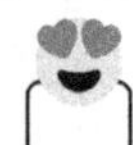 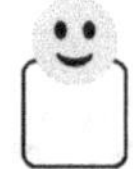 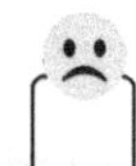 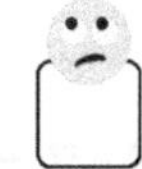 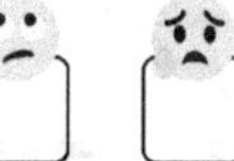 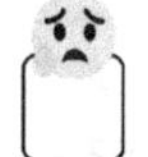

1. Preheat your grill or grill pan to medium-high heat. Season the salmon fillet with salt and pepper, then grill for 4-5 minutes per side, or until cooked through.

2. In a large salad bowl, combine the baby arugula, cooked quinoa, sliced cucumber, crumbled feta cheese, and chopped walnuts.

3. In a small bowl, whisk together the ingredients for the dressing: olive oil, balsamic vinegar, Dijon mustard, honey, and salt and pepper to taste.

4. Flake the grilled salmon into bite-sized pieces and add it to the salad. Drizzle the dressing over the salad and toss gently to coat.

This fertility-boosting grilled salmon salad is packed with nutrients that can help support reproductive health for both men and women:

- Salmon is a rich source of omega-3 fatty acids, which can help improve sperm quality and support overall fertility.
- Arugula is a nutrient-dense green that's high in folate, antioxidants, and minerals like iron, which are important for egg and sperm health.
- Quinoa is a complete protein source that also provides fiber, B vitamins, and minerals like magnesium, which can help regulate hormones and support fertility.
- Cucumber is hydrating and contains vitamins and minerals that can help reduce inflammation and support overall reproductive function.
- Feta cheese is a good source of protein, calcium, and vitamin B12, all of which can help improve fertility.
- Walnuts are a great source of omega-3 fatty acids and antioxidants that can help boost fertility.
- The olive oil, balsamic vinegar, and honey in the dressing provide healthy fats and natural sweetness that can help balance hormones and support fertility

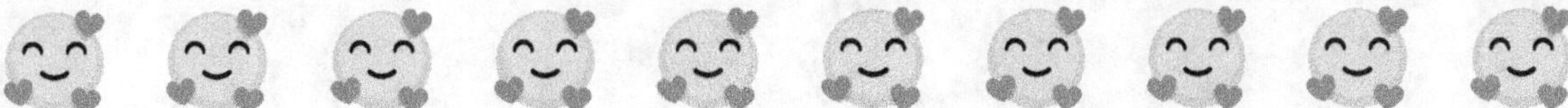

19. Roasted vegetable and farro salad

  Prep Time : Cook Time: 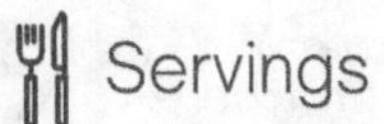 Servings :

Is this dish easy or difficult for you to make?

◯   ◯

Write 5 friends with whom you want to share this dish ....

INGREDIENTS

- 1 cup dry farro, cooked according to package

---

1. Preheat your oven to 400°F (200°C).

2. In a large baking dish, toss the diced butternut squash, zucchini, and red bell pepper with 1 tbsp of olive oil. Season with salt and pepper.

3. Roast the vegetables in the preheated oven for 20-25 minutes, or until they are tender and lightly browned.

4. In a large salad bowl, combine the cooked farro, roasted vegetables, baby spinach, crumbled feta cheese, and chopped walnuts.

5. In a small bowl, whisk together the ingredients for the dressing: olive oil, balsamic vinegar, Dijon mustard, honey, and salt and pepper to taste. Drizzle the dressing over the salad and toss gently to coat.

This fertility-boosting roasted vegetable and farro salad is packed with nutrients that can help support reproductive health for both men and women:

- Farro is a whole grain that's high in fiber, protein, and B vitamins, which are important for fertility.
- Butternut squash, zucchini, and red bell pepper are rich in antioxidants, vitamins, and minerals that can help improve egg and sperm quality.
- Spinach is a great source of folate, iron, and antioxidants, which are crucial for fertility.
- Feta cheese is a good source of protein, calcium, and vitamin B12, all of which can help improve fertility.
- Walnuts are a great source of omega-3 fatty acids and antioxidants that can help regulate hormones and boost fertility.
- The olive oil, balsamic vinegar, and honey in the dressing provide healthy fats and natural sweetness that can help balance hormones and support fertility.

How would you rate this dish?

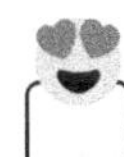  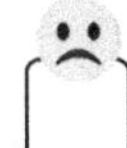 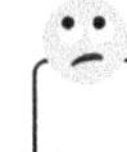 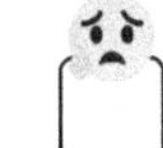

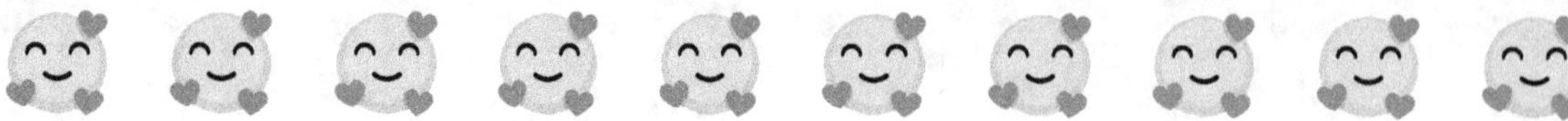

20. Hummus and vegetable wrap with whole-grain tortilla

 Prep Time :   Cook Time :   Servings :

Is this dish easy or difficult for you to make?

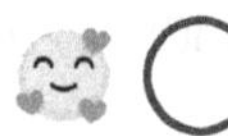 ◯   ◯

Write 5 ....
friends
with   ....
whom
you   ....
want to
share   ....
this
dish   ....

INGREDIENTS

- 1 whole-grain tortilla or wrap
- 2 tbsp hummus
- 1/2 cup sliced cucumber
- 1/2 cup sliced bell pepper
- 1/4 cup shredded carrots
- 1/4 cup baby spinach leaves
- 1 tbsp crumbled feta cheese
- Salt and pepper to taste

1. Lay the whole-grain tortilla or wrap on a flat surface.

2. Spread the hummus evenly over the center of the tortilla.

3. Layer the sliced cucumber, bell pepper, shredded carrots, and baby spinach leaves on top of the hummus.

4. Sprinkle the crumbled feta cheese over the vegetables.

5. Season with salt and pepper to taste.

6. Fold the bottom of the tortilla up over the filling, then fold in the sides and continue rolling tightly to create a wrap.

This fertility-boosting hummus and vegetable wrap is packed with nutrients that can help support reproductive health for both men and women:

- Whole-grain tortilla provides complex carbohydrates, fiber, and B vitamins, which are important for fertility.
- Hummus is a nutritious spread that provides protein, fiber, and healthy fats to support fertility.
- Cucumber is hydrating and contains vitamins and minerals that can help reduce inflammation and support overall reproductive function.
- Bell pepper is a good source of vitamin C, an antioxidant that can help protect against oxidative stress and support fertility.
- Carrots are rich in beta-carotene, which can help improve egg and sperm quality.
- Spinach is a great source of folate, iron, and antioxidants, which are important for egg and sperm health.
- Feta cheese is a good source of protein, calcium, and vitamin B12, all of which can help improve fertility.

How would you rate this dish?

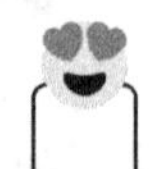 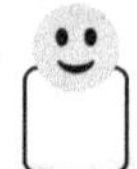 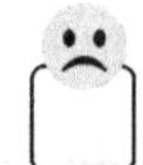 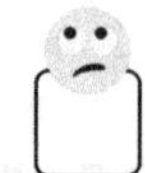 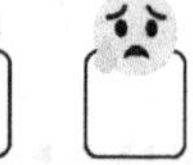

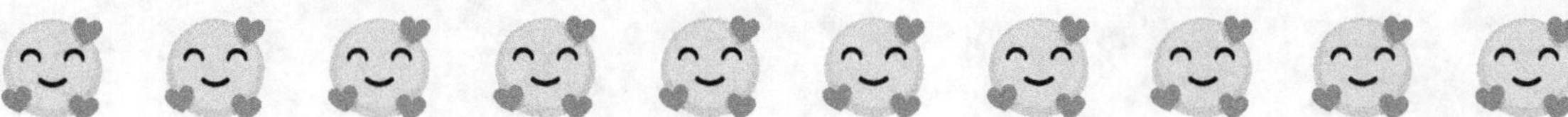

21. Baked salmon with quinoa and steamed broccoli

Prep Time :  Cook Time : Servings :

Is this dish easy or difficult for you to make?

◯   ◯

Write 5 friends with whom you want to share this dish

....
....
....
....
....

INGREDIENTS

- 4 oz salmon fillet
- 1/2 cup cooked quinoa
- 1 cup steamed broccoli florets
- 1 tbsp olive oil
- 1 tsp lemon juice
- 1 tsp Dijon mustard
- Salt and pepper to taste

1. Preheat your oven to 400°F (200°C).

2. Place the salmon fillet on a baking sheet lined with parchment paper. Drizzle with 1 tsp of olive oil and season with salt and pepper.

3. Bake the salmon in the preheated oven for 12-15 minutes, or until it flakes easily with a fork.

4. In a small bowl, whisk together the remaining 2 tsp of olive oil, lemon juice, and Dijon mustard. Season with salt and pepper to taste.

5. In a serving bowl, place the cooked quinoa and steamed broccoli florets.

6. Flake the baked salmon into the bowl with the quinoa and broccoli.

7. Drizzle the lemon-Dijon dressing over the top and gently toss to combine.

This fertility-boosting baked salmon with quinoa and broccoli is packed with nutrients that can help support reproductive health for both men and women:

- Salmon is a rich source of omega-3 fatty acids, which can help improve sperm quality and support overall fertility.
- Quinoa is a complete protein source that also provides fiber, B vitamins, and minerals like magnesium, which can help regulate hormones and support fertility.
- Broccoli is a cruciferous vegetable that's high in folate, antioxidants, and indole-3-carbinol, which can help improve egg and sperm quality.
- The lemon juice and Dijon mustard in the dressing provide vitamin C and other beneficial compounds that can help reduce inflammation and support fertility.

How would you rate this dish?

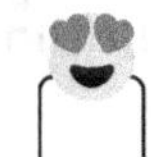 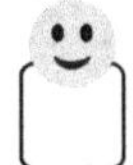 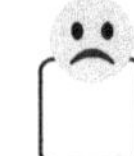 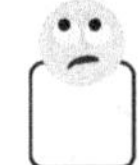 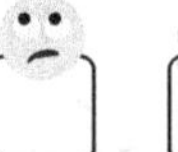 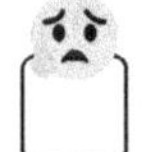

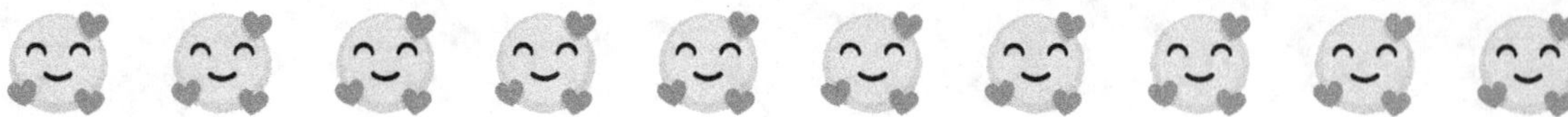

22. Grilled chicken breast with sweet potato and green beans

 Prep Time :    Cook Time :   Servings :

Is this dish easy or difficult for you to make?

😭 ⭕   😊 ⭕

Write 5 friends with whom you want to share this dish

....
....
....
....

INGREDIENTS

- 4 oz boneless, skinless chicken breast
- 1 medium sweet potato, peeled and cubed
- 1 cup fresh green beans, trimmed
- 1 tbsp olive oil
- 1 tsp dried thyme
- Salt and pepper to taste

1. Preheat your grill or grill pan to medium-high heat.

2. Season the chicken breast with salt, pepper, and 1/2 tsp of the dried thyme.

3. Grill the chicken for 5-7 minutes per side, or until it reaches an internal temperature of 165°F (75°C). Set aside and keep warm.

4. In a medium saucepan, bring water to a boil. Add the cubed sweet potato and cook for 8-10 minutes, until tender. Drain and set aside.

5. In the same saucepan, add the green beans and a small amount of water. Steam the green beans for 5-7 minutes, until tender-crisp. Drain and set aside.

6. In a small bowl, whisk together the olive oil and remaining 1/2 tsp of dried thyme.

7. Arrange the grilled chicken, cooked sweet potato, and steamed green beans on a plate. Drizzle the thyme-infused olive oil over the top.

This fertility-boosting grilled chicken with sweet potato and green beans is packed with nutrients that can help support reproductive health for both men and women:

- Chicken is a lean protein source that can help support overall reproductive function.
- Sweet potato is rich in beta-carotene, vitamin C, and other antioxidants that can help improve egg and sperm quality.
- Green beans are a good source of folate, fiber, and other vitamins and minerals that are important for fertility.
- Olive oil and thyme provide healthy fats and anti-inflammatory compounds that can help regulate hormones and support fertility.

How would you rate this dish?

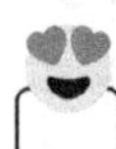 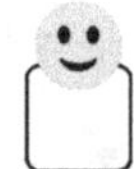 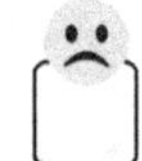 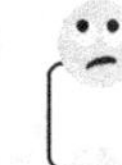 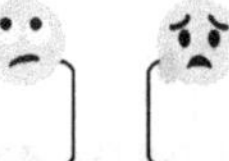 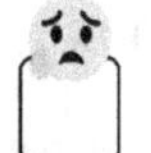

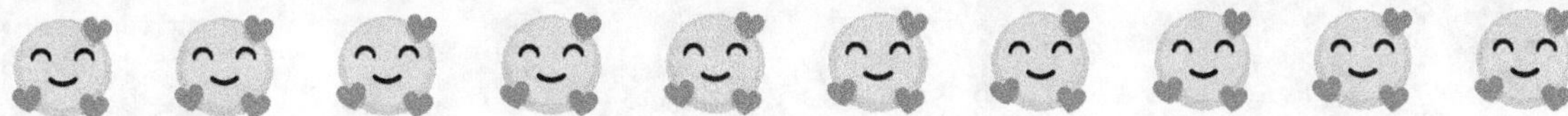

23. Stuffed bell peppers with brown rice and ground turkey

 Prep Time :   Cook Time :   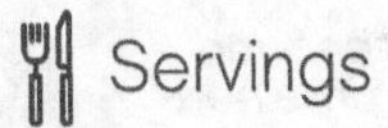 Servings :

Is this dish easy or difficult for you to make?

◯   ◯

Write 5 ....
friends
with   ....
whom
you   ....
want to
share   ....
this
dish   ....

INGREDIENTS

- 4 bell peppers (any color)
- 1 lb ground turkey
- 1 cup cooked brown rice
- 1 small onion, diced
- 2 cloves garlic, minced
- 1 tsp dried oregano
- 1 tsp ground cumin
- 1/4 cup crumbled feta cheese
- Salt and pepper to taste

1. Preheat your oven to 375°F (190°C).

2. Cut the tops off the bell peppers and remove the seeds and membranes. Place the bell pepper shells in a baking dish.

3. In a skillet over medium heat, cook the ground turkey, diced onion, and minced garlic until the turkey is browned and the vegetables are softened, about 5-7 minutes. Drain any excess fat.

4. Stir in the cooked brown rice, dried oregano, and ground cumin. Season with salt and pepper to taste.

5. Spoon the turkey and rice mixture into the hollowed-out bell pepper shells, packing it in tightly.

6. Sprinkle the crumbled feta cheese over the top of the stuffed peppers.

7. Bake the stuffed peppers in the preheated oven for 25-30 minutes, or until the peppers are tender and the filling is hot.

This fertility-boosting stuffed bell pepper dish is packed with nutrients that can help support reproductive health for both men and women:

- Ground turkey is a lean protein source that can help support overall reproductive function.
- Brown rice is a whole grain that provides complex carbohydrates, fiber, and B vitamins, which are important for fertility.
- Bell peppers are rich in vitamin C, an antioxidant that can help protect against oxidative stress and support fertility.
- Onions and garlic contain sulfur-containing compounds that can help improve sperm motility and quality.
- Oregano and cumin are herbs that have been shown to have fertility-enhancing properties.

How would you rate this dish?

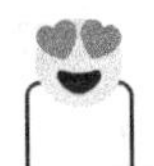 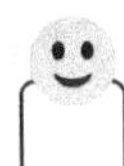 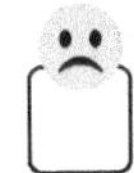 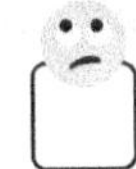 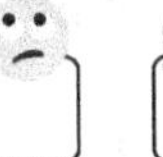 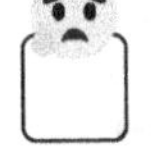

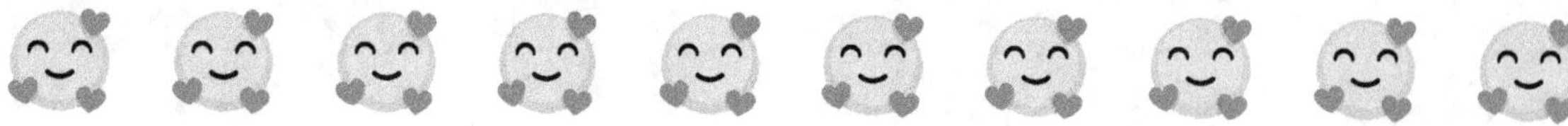

24. Shrimp stir-fry with mixed vegetables and brown rice

 Prep Time : 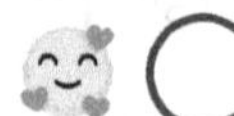 Cook Time : Servings :

Is this dish easy or difficult for you to make?

Write 5 friends with whom you want to share this dish

....
....
....
....
....

INGREDIENTS

- 1 lb shrimp, peeled and deveined
- 2 tbsp sesame oil
- 2 cloves garlic, minced
- 1 inch piece fresh ginger, grated
- 1 cup mixed vegetables (such as broccoli, bell peppers, snow peas, and carrots), chopped
- 2 cups cooked brown rice
- 2 tbsp low-sodium soy sauce
- 1 tsp honey
- Salt and pepper to taste
- Chopped green onions for garnish (optional)

1. Heat the sesame oil in a large skillet or wok over medium-high heat.

2. Add the minced garlic and grated ginger to the hot oil and cook for 1 minute, until fragrant.

3. Add the shrimp to the skillet and stir-fry for 2-3 minutes, until the shrimp start to turn pink.

4. Add the chopped mixed vegetables to the skillet and continue stir-frying for 3-5 minutes, until the vegetables are tender-crisp.

5. Stir in the cooked brown rice, soy sauce, and honey. Season with salt and pepper to taste.

6. Cook for an additional 2-3 minutes, until everything is heated through. Serve the shrimp stir-fry hot, garnished with chopped green onions if desired.

This fertility-boosting shrimp stir-fry is packed with nutrients that can help support reproductive health for both men and women:

- Shrimp is a good source of protein, selenium, and zinc, which are important for fertility.
- Mixed vegetables like broccoli, bell peppers, and carrots are rich in antioxidants, vitamins, and minerals that can help improve egg and sperm quality.
- Brown rice provides complex carbohydrates, fiber, and B vitamins, which are important for overall reproductive function.
- Garlic and ginger contain compounds that can help improve sperm motility and quality.
- Soy sauce and honey provide beneficial compounds that can help regulate hormones and support fertility.

Enjoy this delicious and nutritious shrimp stir-fry with brown rice as part of a balanced diet to help support your fertility journey.

How would you rate this dish?

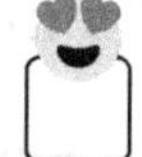 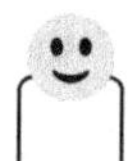 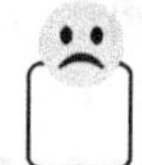 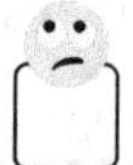 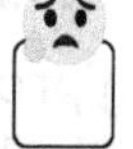

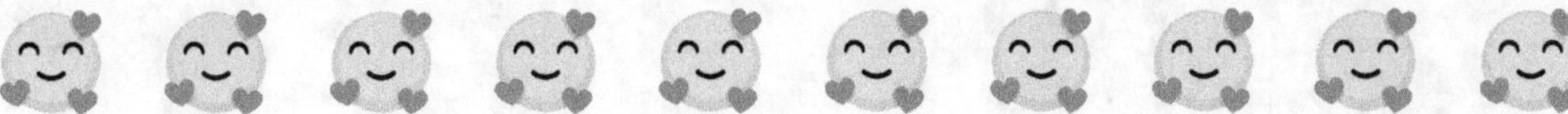

25. Baked cod with a lemon dill sauce and asparagus

Prep Time :   Cook Time :   Servings :

Is this dish easy or difficult for you to make?

 ◯   ◯

Write 5 friends with whom you want to share this dish ....

INGREDIENTS

- 4 (4 oz) cod fillets
- 1 tbsp olive oil
- Salt and pepper to taste
- 1 lb asparagus, trimmed
- Lemon Dill Sauce:
- 1/4 cup plain Greek yogurt
- 2 tbsp fresh lemon juice
- 1 tbsp chopped fresh dill
- 1 tsp Dijon mustard
- 1 garlic clove, minced
- Salt and pepper to taste

1. Preheat your oven to 400°F (200°C).

2. Place the cod fillets in a baking dish and drizzle with the olive oil. Season with salt and pepper.

3. Arrange the trimmed asparagus spears around the cod fillets.

4. Bake the cod and asparagus in the preheated oven for 15-18 minutes, or until the cod is opaque and flakes easily with a fork.

5. While the cod and asparagus are baking, prepare the lemon dill sauce. In a small bowl, whisk together the Greek yogurt, lemon juice, chopped dill, Dijon mustard, and minced garlic. Season with salt and pepper to taste.

6. Serve the baked cod and asparagus warm, with the lemon dill sauce drizzled over the top.

This fertility-boosting baked cod dish is packed with nutrients that can help support reproductive health for both men and women:
- Cod is a lean protein source that's rich in omega-3 fatty acids, which can help improve sperm quality and support overall fertility.

- Asparagus is a nutrient-dense vegetable that's high in folate, antioxidants, and vitamins that can help improve egg and sperm health.

- Greek yogurt is a good source of protein, calcium, and probiotics, which can help support fertility.

- Lemon juice and dill provide vitamin C and anti-inflammatory compounds that can help regulate hormones and reduce oxidative stress.

- Dijon mustard and garlic contain beneficial compounds that can help improve sperm motility and quality.

How would you rate this dish?

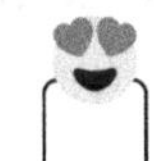 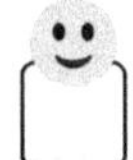 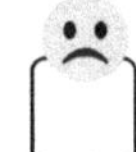 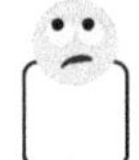 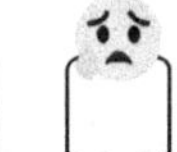

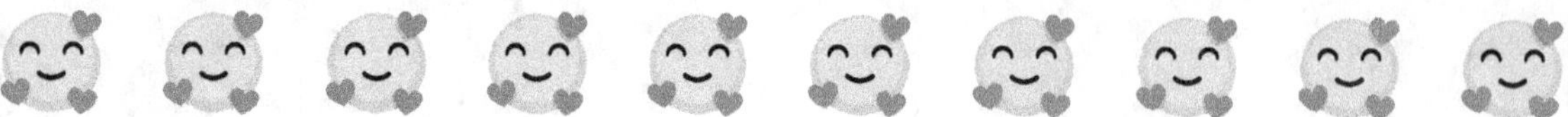

26. Whole-wheat pasta with marinara sauce and turkey meatballs

   Prep Time :   Cook Time :   Servings :

Is this dish easy or difficult for you to make?

 ◯    ◯

Write 5 ....
friends
with   ....
whom
you   ....
want to
share   ....
this
dish   ....

INGREDIENTS

- 8 oz whole-wheat pasta
- 1 lb ground turkey
- 1/4 cup breadcrumbs
- 1 egg
- 2 tbsp grated Parmesan cheese
- 2 cloves garlic, minced
- 1 tsp dried oregano
- Salt and pepper to taste
- 1 jar (24 oz) marinara sauce
- 2 cups baby spinach leaves

1. Bring a large pot of salted water to a boil. Cook the whole-wheat pasta according to package instructions until al dente. Drain and set aside.

2. In a medium bowl, combine the ground turkey, breadcrumbs, egg, Parmesan cheese, minced garlic, and dried oregano. Season with salt and pepper.

3. Roll the turkey mixture into 1-inch meatballs and place them on a baking sheet.

4. Bake the meatballs in a preheated 400°F (200°C) oven for 15-18 minutes, or until cooked through.

5. In a large skillet, heat the marinara sauce over medium heat. Add the cooked whole-wheat pasta and baby spinach leaves to the sauce, tossing to coat.

6. Serve the whole-wheat pasta with the marinara sauce and top with the baked turkey meatballs.

This fertility-boosting whole-wheat pasta dish is packed with nutrients that can help support reproductive health for both men and women:

- Whole-wheat pasta provides complex carbohydrates, fiber, and B vitamins, which are important for fertility.
- Ground turkey is a lean protein source that can help support overall reproductive function.
- Breadcrumbs, Parmesan cheese, and egg help bind the meatballs and provide additional protein and nutrients.
- Garlic and oregano contain compounds that can help improve sperm motility and quality.
- Marinara sauce is a good source of lycopene, an antioxidant that can help protect against oxidative stress and support fertility.
- Baby spinach leaves are rich in folate, iron, and antioxidants, which are crucial for egg and sperm health.

How would you rate this dish?

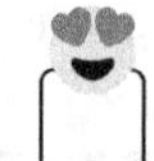 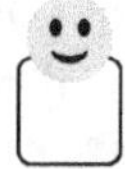 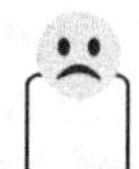 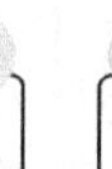 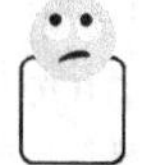 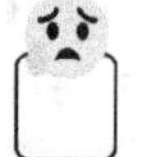

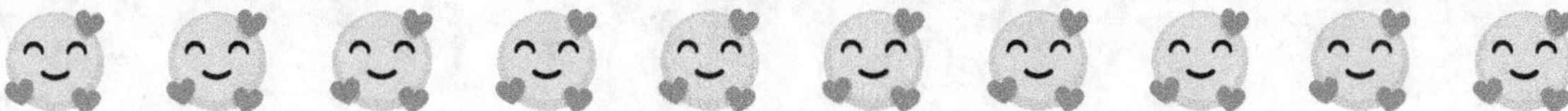

 *Let's do that and fill in the time here* — Prep Time :   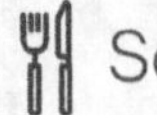 Cook Time :   Servings :

Is this dish easy or difficult for you to make?

○   ○

Write 5 friends with whom you want to share this dish

....

....

....

....

....

INGREDIENTS

- 1 block of firm or extra-firm tofu, cubed
- 2 tbsp oil (such as coconut or vegetable oil)
- 1 onion, diced
- 3 cloves garlic, minced
- 1 tbsp grated ginger
- 2 tsp curry powder
- 1 tsp ground cumin
- 1 tsp ground coriander
- 1 tsp turmeric
- 1 cup diced tomatoes (canned or fresh)
- 1 cup vegetable broth
- 1 cup coconut milk
- 2 cups mixed vegetables (such as bell peppers, cauliflower, spinach, etc.), chopped
- Salt and pepper to taste
- Cooked brown rice, for serving

1. Press the tofu for 15-30 minutes to remove excess moisture. Cut into 1-inch cubes.

2. In a large skillet or wok, heat the oil over medium heat. Add the tofu cubes and cook for 5-7 minutes, turning occasionally, until lightly browned on all sides. Remove tofu from the pan and set aside.

3. In the same pan, sauté the onion for 3-4 minutes until translucent. Add the garlic and ginger and cook for 1 minute more.

4. Stir in the curry powder, cumin, coriander, and turmeric. Cook for 1 minute to toast the spices.

5. Pour in the diced tomatoes, vegetable broth, and coconut milk. Bring to a simmer.

6. Add the chopped vegetables and the cooked tofu. Simmer for 10-15 minutes, until the vegetables are tender.

7. Season with salt and pepper to taste.

8. Serve the curry over cooked brown rice.

Enjoy your flavorful and nutritious tofu and vegetable curry!

How would you rate this dish?

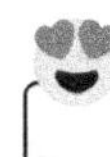 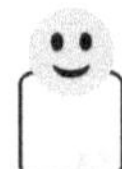  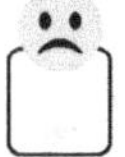 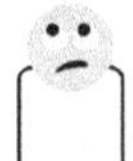 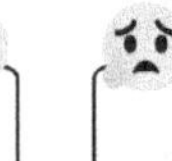

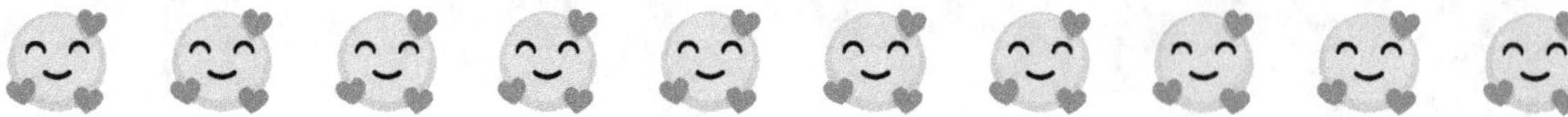

28. Grilled steak with a side of roasted Brussels sprouts

 Prep Time :   Cook Time :   Servings :

Is this dish easy or difficult for you to make?

○   ○

Write 5 ....
friends
with ....
whom
you ....
want to
share ....
this
dish ....

INGREDIENTS

Steak:
- 2 lbs flank or skirt steak
- 2 tbsp olive oil
- 2 tsp garlic powder
- 1 tsp onion powder
- Salt and pepper to taste

Brussels Sprouts:
- 1 lb Brussels sprouts, trimmed and halved
- 2 tbsp olive oil
- 1 tsp balsamic vinegar
- Salt and pepper to taste

Steak:
1. Pat the steak dry with paper towels and season generously with the garlic powder, onion powder, salt, and pepper.

2. Heat a grill or grill pan over high heat. Brush the steak with olive oil.

3. Grill the steak for 3-5 minutes per side, depending on thickness, until it reaches your desired doneness.

4. Let the steak rest for 5-10 minutes before slicing against the grain.

Brussels Sprouts:
1. Preheat the oven to 400°F.

2. Toss the Brussels sprouts with the olive oil, balsamic vinegar, salt, and pepper.

3. Spread the Brussels sprouts in a single layer on a baking sheet.

4. Roast for 20-25 minutes, tossing halfway, until the Brussels sprouts are tender and lightly browned.

Fertility-Boosting Benefits:
- Steak is a good source of protein, iron, and zinc, which are important for fertility in both men and women.
- Brussels sprouts are rich in folate, a nutrient essential for fetal development and reducing the risk of birth defects.
- The combination of protein, vegetables, and healthy fats in this meal can help support overall reproductive health for couples trying to conceive.

Serve the grilled steak with the roasted Brussels sprouts for a delicious and fertility-friendly meal.

How would you rate this dish?

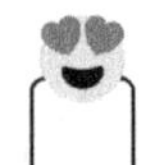 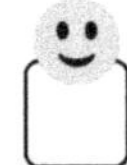 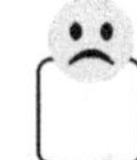 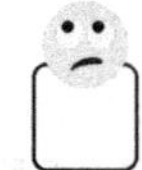 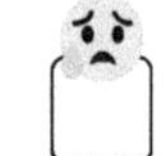

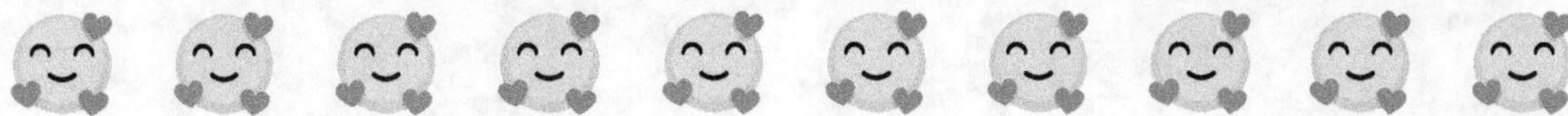

29. Lamb chops with mint yogurt sauce and roasted carrots

 Prep Time :   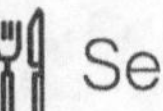 Cook Time :   Servings :

Is this dish easy or difficult for you to make?

 ◯   ◯

Write 5 friends with whom you want to share this dish ....

INGREDIENTS

Lamb Chops:
- 4 lamb chops (about 1-1.5 lbs total)
- 2 tbsp olive oil
- Salt and pepper to taste

Mint Yogurt Sauce:
- 1 cup plain Greek yogurt
- 2 tbsp chopped fresh mint
- 1 tbsp lemon juice
- 1 garlic clove, minced
- Salt and pepper to taste

Roasted Carrots:
- 1 lb carrots, peeled and cut into 1-inch pieces
- 2 tbsp olive oil
- 1 tsp ground cumin
- Salt and pepper to taste

1. Preheat the oven to 400°F.

Roasted Carrots:
1. Toss the carrot pieces with the olive oil, cumin, salt, and pepper.

2. Spread the carrots in a single layer on a baking sheet.

3. Roast for 20-25 minutes, tossing halfway, until the carrots are tender and lightly browned.

Lamb Chops:
1. Season the lamb chops generously with salt and pepper.

2. Heat the olive oil in a large skillet over medium-high heat.

3. Add the lamb chops and cook for 3-4 minutes per side, or until they reach your desired doneness.

4. Let the lamb chops rest for 5 minutes before serving.

Mint Yogurt Sauce:
1. In a small bowl, mix together the Greek yogurt, chopped mint, lemon juice, garlic, salt, and pepper.

To Serve:
1. Place the lamb chops on a plate and top with the mint yogurt sauce.

2. Serve the roasted carrots on the side.

Enjoy this flavorful and nutritious lamb chop dish with the refreshing mint yogurt sauce and roasted carrots.

How would you rate this dish?

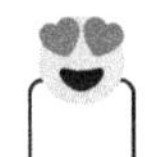 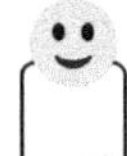  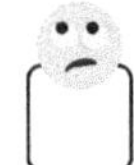 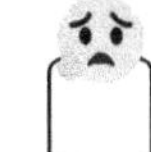

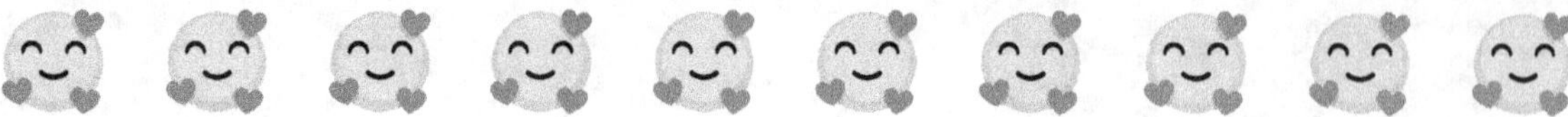

30. Chicken and vegetable kabobs with a side of quinoa

Let's do that and fill in the time here

Prep Time :

Cook Time :

Servings :

Is this dish easy or difficult for you to make?

○   ○

Write 5 friends with whom you want to share this dish

....

....

....

....

....

INGREDIENTS

Kabobs:
- 1 lb boneless, skinless chicken breasts, cut into 1-inch cubes
- 1 red bell pepper, cut into 1-inch pieces
- 1 yellow bell pepper, cut into 1-inch pieces
- 1 red onion, cut into 1-inch pieces
- 8 oz mushrooms, halved
- 2 tbsp olive oil
- 1 tsp dried oregano
- 1 tsp garlic powder
- Salt and pepper to taste

Quinoa:
- 1 cup quinoa, rinsed
- 2 cups low-sodium chicken or vegetable broth
- 1 tbsp chopped fresh parsley

Kabobs:
1. Preheat the grill or grill pan to medium-high heat.

2. In a large bowl, toss the chicken, bell peppers, onion, and mushrooms with the olive oil, oregano, garlic powder, salt, and pepper until well coated.

3. Thread the chicken and vegetables onto skewers, alternating the ingredients.

4. Grill the kabobs for 12-15 minutes, turning occasionally, until the chicken is cooked through and the vegetables are tender.

Quinoa:
1. In a medium saucepan, combine the quinoa and broth. Bring to a boil over high heat.

2. Reduce the heat to low, cover, and simmer for 15-20 minutes, or until the quinoa is tender and the liquid is absorbed.

3. Fluff the quinoa with a fork and stir in the chopped parsley.

To Serve:
1. Serve the grilled chicken and vegetable kabobs over the cooked quinoa.

This dish is a great source of lean protein, fiber, and a variety of vitamins and minerals. The quinoa provides a nutritious base, while the kabobs offer a flavorful and colorful main course.

How would you rate this dish?

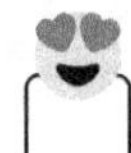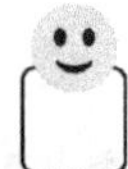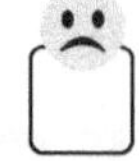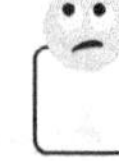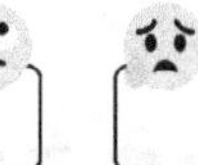

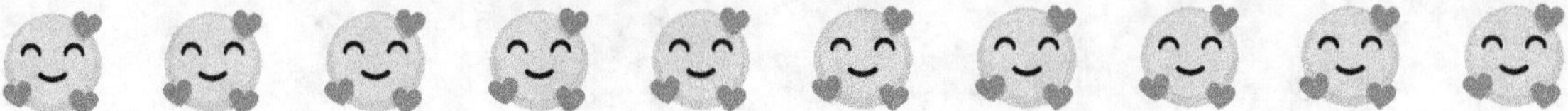

31. Mixed nuts (almonds, walnuts, cashews)

Prep Time :　　Cook Time :　　Servings :

Is this dish easy or difficult for you to make?

 ◯　　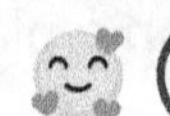 ◯

Write 5 friends with whom you want to share this dish

....

....

....

....

....

INGREDIENTS

- 1 cup raw almonds
- 1 cup raw walnuts
- 1 cup raw cashews

1. Preheat oven to 350°F (175°C).

2. Spread the almonds, walnuts, and cashews out in a single layer on a baking sheet.

3. Roast the nuts for 8-10 minutes, stirring halfway, until lightly golden and fragrant.

4. Remove the nuts from the oven and let cool completely.

5. Once cooled, transfer the mixed nuts to an airtight container.

6. Store the mixed nuts at room temperature for up to 2 weeks.

You can adjust the ratios of the different nuts to your preference. The key is to roast them together to bring out their natural flavors. Enjoy these crunchy, protein-packed mixed nuts as a snack or use them in salads, baked goods, or other recipes.

How would you rate this dish?

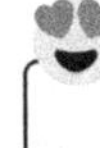   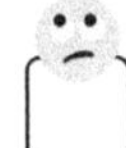 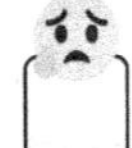

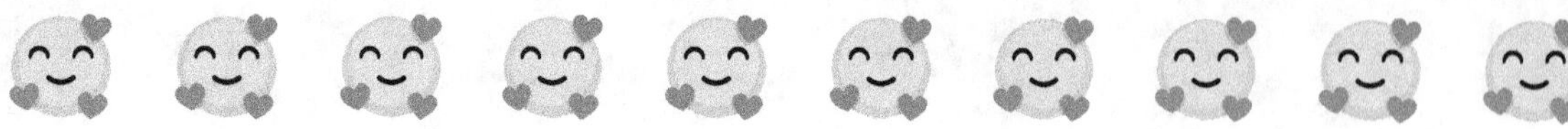

32. Apple slices with almond butter

Prep Time :   Cook Time :   Servings :

Is this dish easy or difficult for you to make?

 ◯   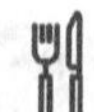 ◯

Write 5 ....
friends
with   ....
whom
you   ....
want to
share   ....
this
dish   ....

INGREDIENTS

- 2 medium apples, cored and sliced
- 1/4 cup all-natural almond butter

For Fertility Support:
- 1 tbsp ground flaxseed
- 1 tsp cinnamon
- 1 tsp honey (optional)

1. Arrange the apple slices on a plate or platter.

2. In a small bowl, mix together the almond butter, ground flaxseed, and cinnamon until well combined.

3. Drizzle the almond butter mixture over the apple slices.

4. If desired, drizzle a small amount of honey over the top.

The key fertility-supporting ingredients in this recipe are:

- Almonds: Rich in healthy fats, protein, and antioxidants that support reproductive health.
- Flaxseed: High in omega-3s and lignans that can help balance hormones.
- Cinnamon: May help regulate menstrual cycles and improve fertility.

This simple snack provides a nutritious combination of fiber, healthy fats, and fertility-boosting nutrients. It's a great option for couples trying to conceive. Enjoy!

How would you rate this dish?

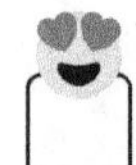 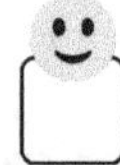 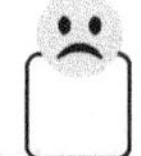 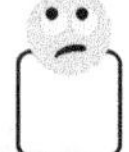 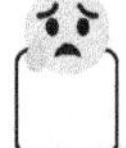

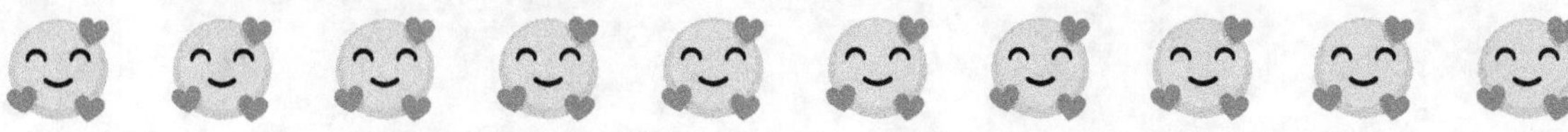

33. Carrot sticks with hummus

Let's do that and fill in the time here

Prep Time : Cook Time : Servings :

Is this dish easy or difficult for you to make?

 ◯   ◯

Write 5 friends with whom you want to share this dish ....

INGREDIENTS

- 4-5 medium carrots, peeled and cut into sticks
- 1 (15 oz) can chickpeas, drained and rinsed
- 2 tbsp tahini
- 2 tbsp lemon juice
- 2 cloves garlic, minced
- 1 tsp ground cumin
- 1/4 tsp cayenne pepper (optional)
- 2 tbsp extra virgin olive oil
- Salt and pepper to taste

For Fertility Support:
- 2 tbsp ground flaxseed
- 1 tbsp raw pumpkin seeds

How would you rate this dish?

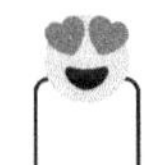 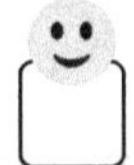 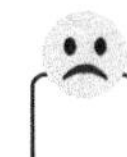  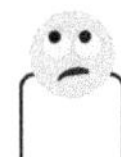 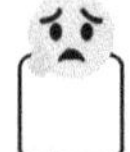

1. In a food processor, combine the chickpeas, tahini, lemon juice, garlic, cumin, cayenne (if using), olive oil, salt, and pepper. Blend until smooth and creamy.

2. Stir in the ground flaxseed and pumpkin seeds until well incorporated.

3. Transfer the hummus to a serving bowl and serve with the carrot sticks for dipping.

The key fertility-supporting ingredients in this recipe are:

- Chickpeas: Rich in folate, zinc, and protein to support reproductive health.

- Tahini: High in calcium, magnesium, and antioxidants.
- Flaxseed: Provides omega-3s and lignans that can help balance hormones.

- Pumpkin seeds: A good source of zinc, which is important for fertility in both men and women.

This nutrient-dense snack provides a satisfying crunch along with a creamy, protein-packed dip. Enjoy this fertility-boosting combo as a healthy snack or appetizer.

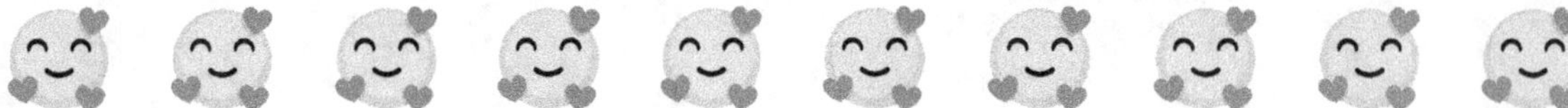

34. Fresh berries with a handful of sunflower seeds

 Prep Time :   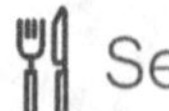 Cook Time :   Servings :

Is this dish easy or difficult for you to make?

😭 ◯   🥰 ◯

Write 5 friends with whom you want to share this dish

....

....

....

....

....

INGREDIENTS

- 1 cup mixed fresh berries (such as strawberries, blueberries, raspberries, blackberries)
- 2 tablespoons raw, unsalted sunflower seeds

For Fertility Support:
- 1 tablespoon ground flaxseed
- 1 teaspoon honey (optional)

1. Rinse and gently pat dry the fresh berries. Place them in a serving bowl.

2. Sprinkle the raw sunflower seeds over the top of the berries.

3. In a small bowl, mix together the ground flaxseed. If desired, drizzle the honey over the top.

4. Serve the berry and sunflower seed mixture immediately.

The key fertility-supporting ingredients in this recipe are:

- Berries: Rich in antioxidants, vitamins, and fiber to support reproductive health.

- Sunflower seeds: High in zinc, selenium, and vitamin E - all important for fertility.

- Flaxseed: Provides omega-3s and lignans that can help balance hormones.

- Honey: Contains antioxidants and may help regulate menstrual cycles.

This simple, nutrient-dense snack is a great option for couples trying to conceive. The combination of fresh berries, crunchy sunflower seeds, and fertility-boosting flaxseed makes it a delicious and healthy choice.

How would you rate this dish?

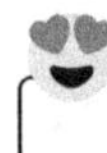 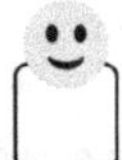 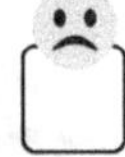 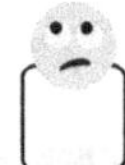 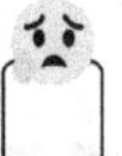

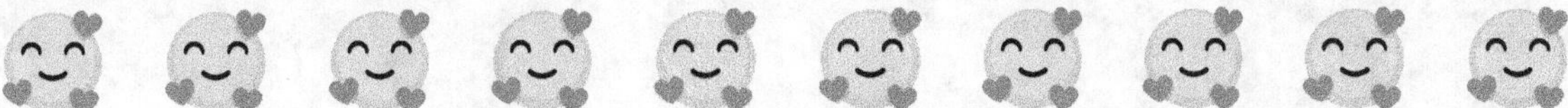

35. Air-popped popcorn with olive oil

  Prep Time :   Cook Time :   Servings :

Is this dish easy or difficult for you to make?

Write 5 friends with whom you want to share this dish

....
....
....
....
....

INGREDIENTS

- 1/2 cup unpopped popcorn kernels
- 1 tbsp extra virgin olive oil
- 1/4 tsp sea salt

For Fertility Support:
- 1 tbsp ground flaxseed
- 1 tsp nutritional yeast
- 1/2 tsp ground turmeric

1. Pop the popcorn kernels using an air popper according to manufacturer's instructions.

2. Transfer the freshly popped popcorn to a large bowl. Drizzle with the olive oil and sprinkle with the sea salt. Toss to coat evenly.

3. In a small bowl, mix together the ground flaxseed, nutritional yeast, and turmeric.

4. Sprinkle the fertility-boosting topping mixture over the popcorn and toss gently to distribute.

The key fertility-supporting ingredients in this recipe are:

- Flaxseed: High in omega-3s and lignans that can help balance hormones.

- Nutritional yeast: A good source of B vitamins, which are important for reproductive health.

- Turmeric: Contains curcumin, an anti-inflammatory compound that may improve fertility.

The healthy fats from the olive oil also help your body absorb the fat-soluble nutrients in this snack. This air-popped popcorn makes a delicious and fertility-supporting treat for couples trying to conceive.

How would you rate this dish?

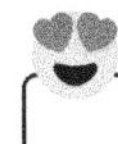 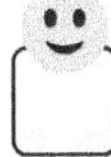 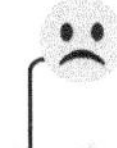 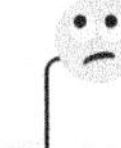 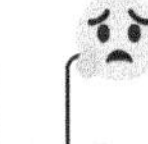 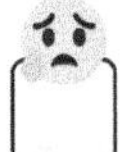

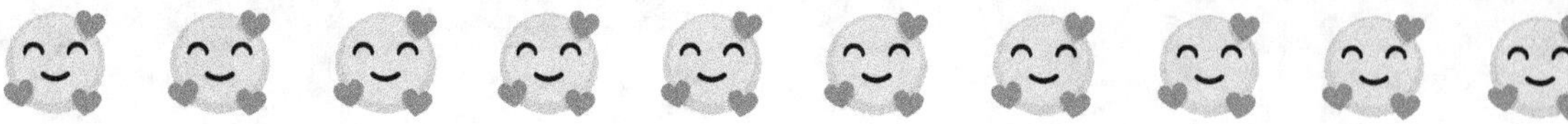

36. Whole-grain crackers with guacamole

 Prep Time :   Cook Time :   Servings :

Is this dish easy or difficult for you to make?

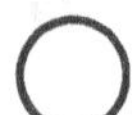 ◯   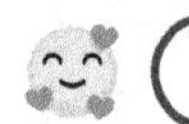 ◯

Write 5 ....
friends
with   ....
whom
you   ....
want to
share   ....
this
dish   ....

INGREDIENTS

For the Guacamole:
- 2 ripe avocados, pitted and mashed
- 1/4 cup diced red onion
- 1 clove garlic, minced
- 1 tbsp fresh lime juice
- 2 tbsp chopped cilantro
- 1/4 tsp sea salt
- 1/4 tsp ground cumin

For Fertility Support:
- 1 tbsp ground flaxseed
- 1 tbsp pumpkin seeds, chopped

For Serving:
- 1 package whole-grain crackers

1. In a medium bowl, mash the avocados with a fork or potato masher.

2. Stir in the red onion, garlic, lime juice, cilantro, salt, and cumin until well combined.

3. Fold in the ground flaxseed and chopped pumpkin seeds.

4. Serve the fertility-boosting guacamole with the whole-grain crackers.

The key fertility-supporting ingredients in this recipe are:

- Avocado: Rich in healthy fats, folate, and antioxidants that support reproductive health.

- Flaxseed: High in omega-3s and lignans that can help balance hormones.

- Pumpkin seeds: A good source of zinc, which is important for fertility in both men and women.

The whole-grain crackers provide a satisfying crunch and complex carbohydrates to round out this nutrient-dense snack. Enjoy this fertility-boosting guacamole and cracker combo as a healthy appetizer or light meal.

How would you rate this dish?

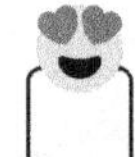 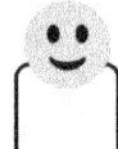 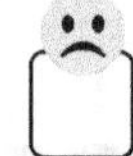 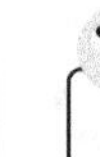 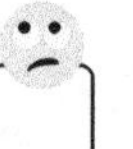 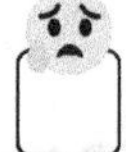

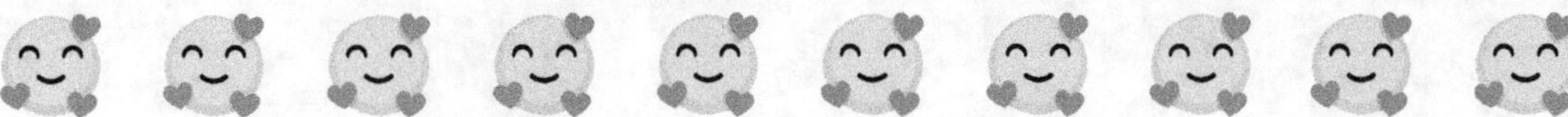

37. Edamame with sea salt

 Prep Time :   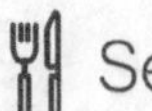 Cook Time :   Servings :

Is this dish easy or difficult for you to make?

😭 ◯   😊 ◯

Write 5 friends with whom you want to share this dish ....

INGREDIENTS

- 1 lb frozen edamame in the pod
- 1 tsp sea salt

For Fertility Support:
- 1 tbsp sesame seeds
- 1 tsp ground ginger

1. Bring a large pot of water to a boil. Add the frozen edamame and cook for 5-7 minutes until tender.

2. Drain the edamame and transfer to a serving bowl.

3. Sprinkle the sea salt over the edamame.

4. In a small bowl, mix together the sesame seeds and ground ginger.

5. Sprinkle the fertility-boosting sesame seed and ginger mixture over the salted edamame.

6. Serve the edamame warm or at room temperature.

The key fertility-supporting ingredients in this recipe are:

- Edamame: Rich in soy isoflavones, protein, and fiber to support reproductive health.

- Sesame seeds: High in zinc, which is important for male and female fertility.

- Ginger: Contains compounds that may help regulate menstrual cycles and improve fertility.

This simple snack provides a satisfying crunch and a boost of fertility-supporting nutrients. The combination of salty edamame, nutty sesame seeds, and warming ginger makes for a delicious and healthy treat for couples trying to conceive.

How would you rate this dish?

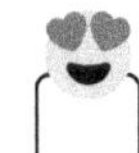  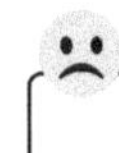 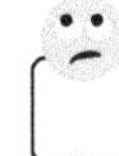 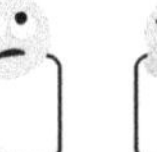 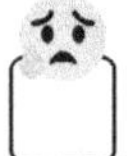

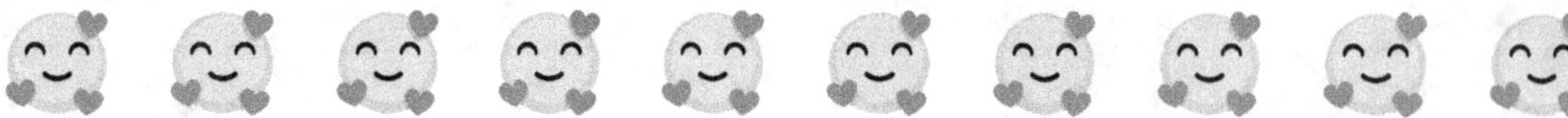

Let's do that and fill in the time here

 Prep Time :   🕐 Cook Time :   🍴 Servings :

Is this dish easy or difficult for you to make?

😭 ◯   🙂 ◯

Write 5 friends with whom you want to share this dish
....
....
....
....
....

INGREDIENTS

- 1 cup plain Greek yogurt
- 1-2 tbsp raw, unprocessed honey
- 1 tsp ground cinnamon

For Fertility Support:
- 1 tbsp ground flaxseed
- 1 tbsp chopped walnuts

1. Scoop the Greek yogurt into a serving bowl.

2. Drizzle the raw honey over the top of the yogurt.

3. Sprinkle the ground cinnamon evenly over the honey-yogurt mixture.

4. In a small bowl, mix together the ground flaxseed and chopped walnuts.

5. Sprinkle the flaxseed-walnut mixture over the top of the yogurt.

The key fertility-supporting ingredients in this recipe are:

- Greek yogurt: High in protein, calcium, and probiotics to support reproductive health.

- Honey: Contains antioxidants and may help regulate menstrual cycles.

- Flaxseed: Rich in omega-3s and lignans that can help balance hormones.

- Walnuts: A good source of omega-3s, zinc, and folate - all important for fertility.

- Cinnamon: May help improve insulin sensitivity and regulate ovulation.

This simple, nutrient-dense snack provides a delicious and fertility-boosting combination of creamy yogurt, sweet honey, and crunchy nuts and seeds. Enjoy this as a healthy breakfast, snack, or dessert.

How would you rate this dish?

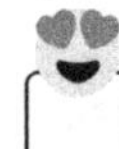 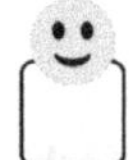 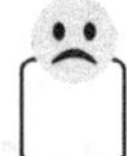 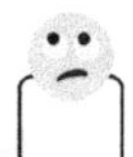 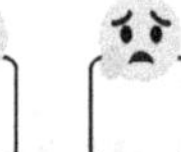

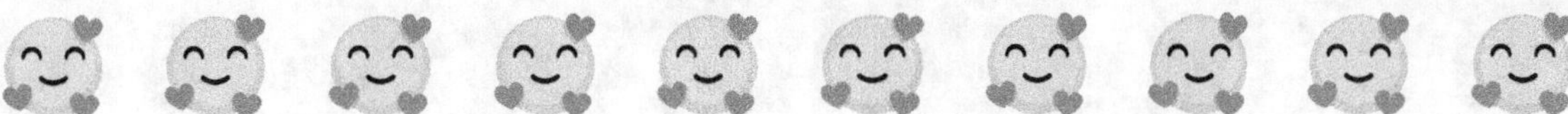

39. Cottage cheese with blueberries

 Prep Time : 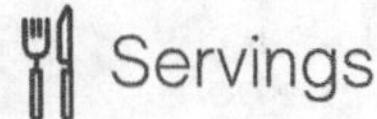 Cook Time : Servings :

Is this dish easy or difficult for you to make?

⭕   ⭕

Write 5 friends with whom you want to share this dish

....
....
....
....
....

INGREDIENTS

- 1 cup low-fat cottage cheese
- 1 cup fresh blueberries
- 1 tbsp honey (optional)

For Fertility Support:
- 1 tbsp ground flaxseed
- 1 tsp cinnamon

1. Scoop the cottage cheese into a serving bowl.

2. Top the cottage cheese with the fresh blueberries.

3. If desired, drizzle the honey over the top.

4. In a small bowl, mix together the ground flaxseed and cinnamon.

5. Sprinkle the flaxseed-cinnamon mixture over the cottage cheese and blueberries.

The key fertility-supporting ingredients in this recipe are:

- Cottage cheese: High in protein, calcium, and probiotics to support reproductive health.

- Blueberries: Rich in antioxidants, vitamins, and fiber that can improve fertility.

- Flaxseed: Provides omega-3s and lignans that can help balance hormones.

- Cinnamon: May help regulate menstrual cycles and improve fertility.

The combination of creamy cottage cheese, sweet blueberries, and fertility-boosting flaxseed and cinnamon makes this a delicious and nutritious snack or light meal. The honey adds a touch of sweetness, but is optional.

This simple dish is a great option for couples trying to conceive, as it provides a nourishing blend of protein, healthy fats, and antioxidants to support reproductive health.

How would you rate this dish?

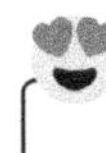   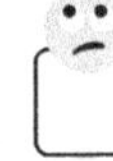 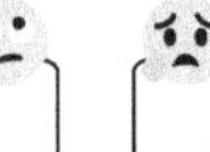

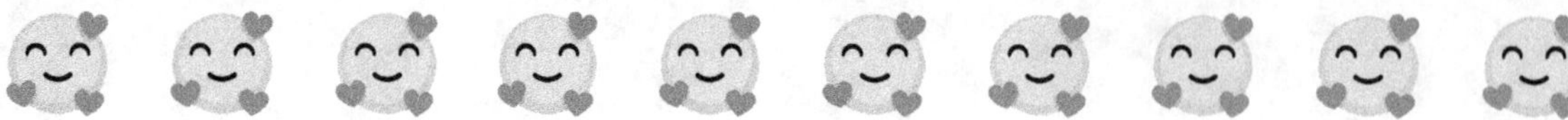

40. Dark chocolate squares with almonds

Let's do that and fill in the time here

Prep Time :   Cook Time :   Servings :

Is this dish easy or difficult for you to make?

 ◯   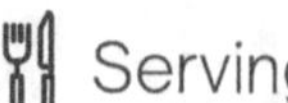 ◯

Write 5 friends with whom you want to share this dish ....

INGREDIENTS

- 2 oz dark chocolate (70% cacao or higher), chopped into squares
- 1/4 cup raw, unsalted almonds

For Fertility Support:
- 1 tbsp ground flaxseed
- 1 tsp cinnamon

1. Arrange the chopped dark chocolate squares on a plate or small platter.

2. Sprinkle the raw almonds over the top of the chocolate.

3. In a small bowl, mix together the ground flaxseed and cinnamon.

4. Sprinkle the flaxseed-cinnamon mixture evenly over the chocolate and almonds.

The key fertility-supporting ingredients in this recipe are:

- Dark chocolate: Rich in antioxidants that can improve blood flow and support reproductive health.

- Almonds: High in healthy fats, protein, and vitamins that are important for fertility.

- Flaxseed: Provides omega-3s and lignans that can help balance hormones.

- Cinnamon: May help regulate menstrual cycles and improve fertility.

This simple, indulgent snack provides a delicious way to get a boost of fertility-supporting nutrients. The combination of rich dark chocolate, crunchy almonds, and the added benefits of flaxseed and cinnamon make this a great treat for couples trying to conceive.

Enjoy these dark chocolate squares in moderation as part of a balanced, fertility-friendly diet.

How would you rate this dish?

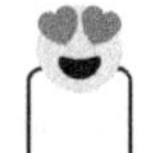 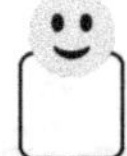  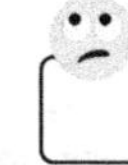 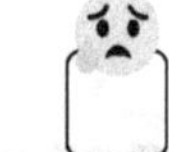

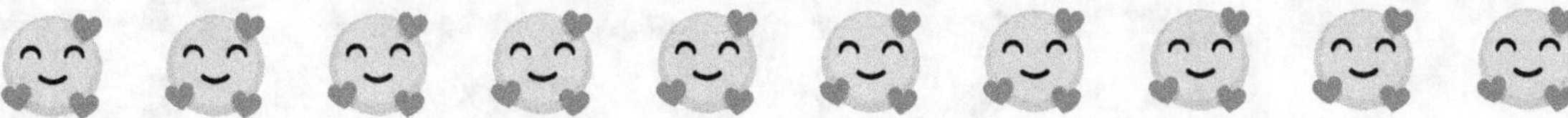

41. Tomato basil soup with a side of whole-grain bread

Let's do that and fill in the time here

 Prep Time :   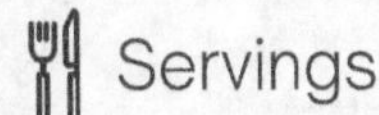 Cook Time :   Servings :

Is this dish easy or difficult for you to make?

Write 5 friends with whom you want to share this dish ....

INGREDIENTS

- 1 tbsp olive oil
- 1 onion, diced
- 3 cloves garlic, minced
- 1 (28 oz) can diced tomatoes
- 2 cups vegetable or chicken broth
- 1/4 cup fresh basil, chopped
- 1 tsp dried oregano
- Salt and pepper to taste

For Fertility Support:
- 2 tbsp ground flaxseed
- 1 tbsp pumpkin seeds, chopped

For Serving:
- Slices of whole-grain bread

1. In a large pot, heat the olive oil over medium heat. Add the onion and sauté for 5 minutes until translucent.

2. Add the garlic and sauté for 1 minute until fragrant.

3. Pour in the diced tomatoes and broth. Stir in the basil and oregano. Season with salt and pepper.

4. Bring the soup to a simmer and let it cook for 10-15 minutes.

5. Remove from heat and use an immersion blender to puree the soup until smooth.

6. Stir in the ground flaxseed and chopped pumpkin seeds.

7. Serve the tomato basil soup warm, with slices of whole-grain bread on the side.

The key fertility-supporting ingredients in this recipe are:

- Tomatoes: Rich in lycopene, an antioxidant that may improve sperm quality and female fertility.

- Basil: Contains compounds that may help regulate menstrual cycles.

- Flaxseed: High in omega-3s and lignans that can help balance hormones.

- Pumpkin seeds: A good source of zinc, which is important for male and female fertility.

The whole-grain bread provides complex carbohydrates to round out this nourishing, fertility-boosting meal. Enjoy this comforting soup as a light lunch or dinner.

How would you rate this dish?

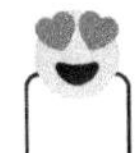 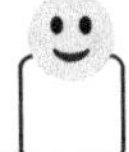 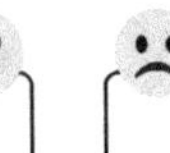  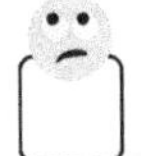 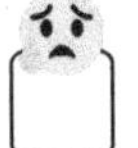

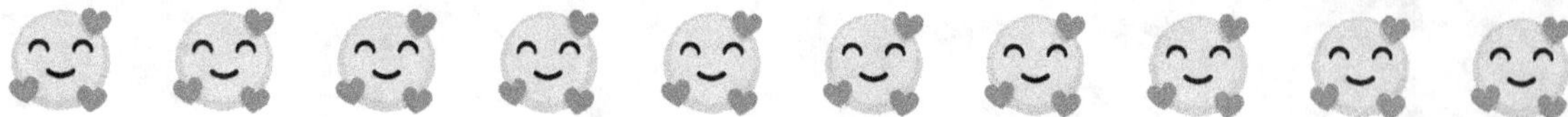

42. Minestrone soup with beans and whole-grain pasta

 Prep Time :   Cook Time :   Servings :

Is this dish easy or difficult for you to make?

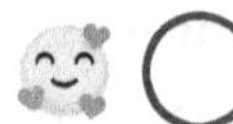 ◯   ◯

Write 5 ....
friends
with   ....
whom
you   ....
want to
share   ....
this
dish   ....

INGREDIENTS

- 1 tbsp olive oil
- 1 onion, diced
- 3 cloves garlic, minced
- 2 carrots, peeled and diced
- 2 celery stalks, diced
- 1 zucchini, diced
- 1 (15 oz) can diced tomatoes
- 4 cups vegetable or chicken broth
- 1 (15 oz) can kidney beans, rinsed and drained
- 1 cup whole-grain elbow macaroni
- 2 cups chopped kale or spinach
- 2 tbsp chopped fresh basil
- Salt and pepper to taste

For Fertility Support:
- 2 tbsp ground flaxseed
- 1 tbsp pumpkin seeds, chopped

How would you rate this dish?

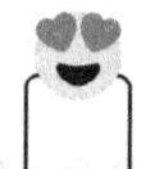 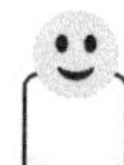 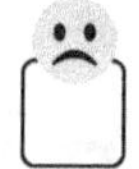 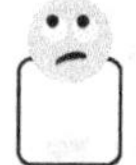 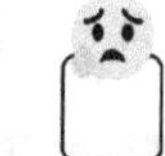

1. In a large pot, heat the olive oil over medium heat. Add the onion and sauté for 5 minutes until translucent.

2. Add the garlic, carrots, celery, and zucchini. Sauté for 3-4 minutes.

3. Pour in the diced tomatoes and broth. Stir in the kidney beans and pasta.

4. Bring the soup to a boil, then reduce heat and simmer for 10-12 minutes, until the pasta is tender.

5. Stir in the kale/spinach and basil. Season with salt and pepper.

6. Remove from heat and stir in the ground flaxseed and chopped pumpkin seeds. Serve the minestrone soup hot.

The key fertility-supporting ingredients in this recipe are:

- Beans: Rich in protein, fiber, and folate to support reproductive health.

- Whole-grain pasta: Provides complex carbs and B vitamins important for fertility.

- Flaxseed: High in omega-3s and lignans that can help balance hormones.

- Pumpkin seeds: A good source of zinc, which is crucial for male and female fertility.

This hearty, nutrient-dense soup is a great option for couples trying to conceive. The combination of vegetables, beans, whole grains, and fertility-boosting seeds and nuts makes it a nourishing and delicious meal.

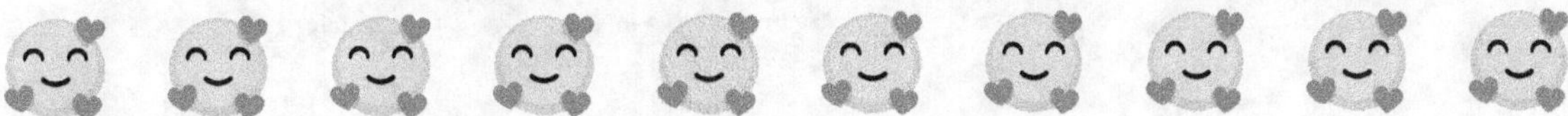

43. Butternut squash soup with a sprinkle of pumpkin seeds

 Prep Time :

Cook Time :

Servings :

Is this dish easy or difficult for you to make?

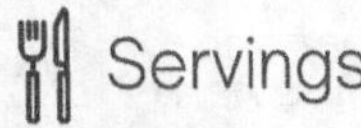

Write 5 friends with whom you want to share this dish

....

....

....

....

....

INGREDIENTS

- 1 medium butternut squash, peeled, seeded, and cubed (about 4 cups)
- 1 onion, diced
- 2 cloves garlic, minced
- 4 cups vegetable or chicken broth
- 1 tsp ground cumin
- 1/2 tsp ground cinnamon
- Salt and pepper to taste
- 2 tbsp pumpkin seeds

1. In a large pot, sauté the onion in a drizzle of olive oil over medium heat for 5 minutes until translucent.

2. Add the garlic and sauté for 1 minute until fragrant.

3. Add the cubed butternut squash and broth. Bring to a boil, then reduce heat and simmer for 20-25 minutes, until the squash is very soft.

4. Remove from heat and use an immersion blender to puree the soup until smooth.

5. Stir in the ground cumin and cinnamon. Season with salt and pepper to taste.

6. Ladle the butternut squash soup into bowls and sprinkle the pumpkin seeds over the top.

The pumpkin seeds add a delightful crunch and a boost of fertility-supporting nutrients to this creamy, comforting soup. Pumpkin seeds are a great source of zinc, which is important for both male and female fertility.

This simple, nourishing soup makes a wonderful appetizer or light meal. Enjoy it as part of a balanced, fertility-friendly diet.

How would you rate this dish?

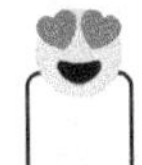 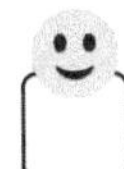  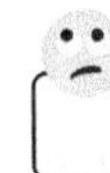 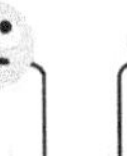 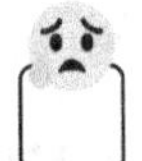

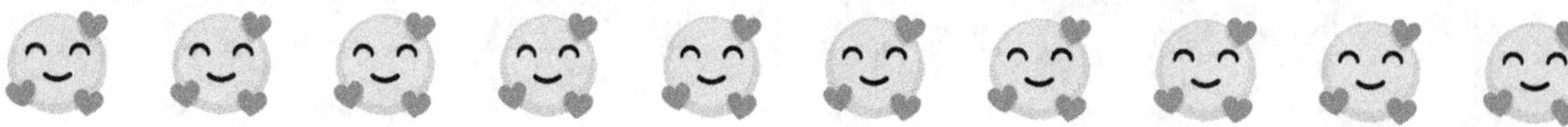

44. Split pea soup with carrots and celery

 Prep Time :   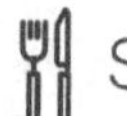 Cook Time :   Servings :

Is this dish easy or difficult for you to make?

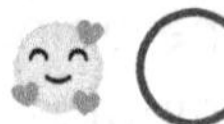 ◯   ◯

Write 5 ....
friends
with ....
whom
you ....
want to
share ....
this
dish ....

INGREDIENTS

- 1 tbsp olive oil
- 1 onion, diced
- 3 cloves garlic, minced
- 2 carrots, peeled and diced
- 2 celery stalks, diced
- 1 lb dried split peas, rinsed
- 6 cups vegetable or chicken broth
- 1 bay leaf
- 1 tsp dried thyme
- Salt and pepper to taste

For Fertility Support:
- 2 tbsp ground flaxseed
- 1 tbsp chopped walnuts

How would you rate this dish?

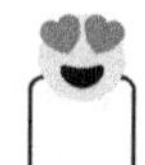 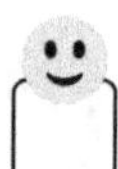 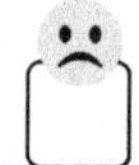 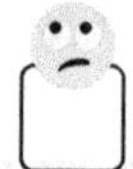 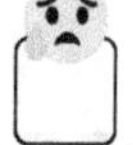

1. In a large pot, heat the olive oil over medium heat. Add the onion and sauté for 5 minutes until translucent.

2. Add the garlic, carrots, and celery. Sauté for 3-4 minutes.

3. Stir in the split peas, broth, bay leaf, and thyme. Season with salt and pepper.

4. Bring the soup to a boil, then reduce heat and simmer for 45-60 minutes, stirring occasionally, until the peas are very soft.

5. Remove the bay leaf. Use an immersion blender to partially puree the soup, leaving some texture.

6. Stir in the ground flaxseed and chopped walnuts. Serve the split pea soup hot.

The key fertility-supporting ingredients in this recipe are:

- Split peas: High in protein, fiber, and folate to support reproductive health.

- Carrots: Rich in beta-carotene, an antioxidant that may improve sperm quality.

- Flaxseed: Provides omega-3s and lignans that can help balance hormones.

- Walnuts: A good source of omega-3s, zinc, and folate - all important for fertility.

This hearty, nutrient-dense soup is a great option for couples trying to conceive. The combination of fiber-rich split peas, vitamin-packed vegetables, and fertility-boosting seeds and nuts makes it a nourishing and delicious meal.

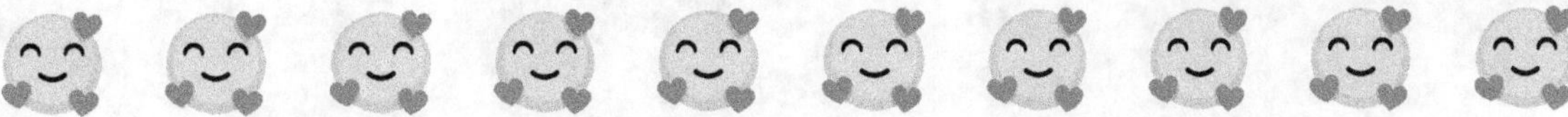

45. Chicken and vegetable soup with quinoa

 Prep Time :   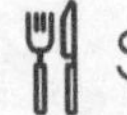 Cook Time :   Servings :

Is this dish easy or difficult for you to make?

Write 5 friends with whom you want to share this dish ....

INGREDIENTS

- 1 tbsp olive oil
- 1 onion, diced
- 3 cloves garlic, minced
- 2 carrots, peeled and diced
- 2 celery stalks, diced
- 1 lb boneless, skinless chicken breasts, cubed
- 6 cups low-sodium chicken broth
- 1 cup cooked quinoa
- 2 cups chopped kale or spinach
- 2 tbsp chopped fresh parsley
- Salt and pepper to taste

For Fertility Support:
- 2 tbsp ground flaxseed
- 1 tbsp pumpkin seeds, chopped

How would you rate this dish?

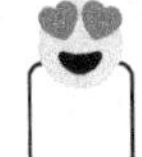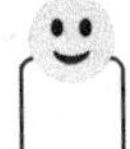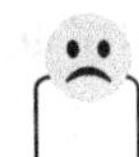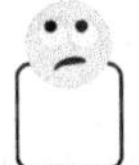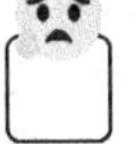

1. In a large pot, heat the olive oil over medium heat. Add the onion and sauté for 5 minutes until translucent.

2. Add the garlic, carrots, and celery. Sauté for 3-4 minutes.

3. Add the cubed chicken and sauté for 2-3 minutes until lightly browned.

4. Pour in the chicken broth and bring to a boil. Reduce heat and simmer for 15-20 minutes, until the chicken is cooked through.

5. Stir in the cooked quinoa, kale/spinach, and parsley. Season with salt and pepper.

6. Remove from heat and stir in the ground flaxseed and chopped pumpkin seeds. Serve the chicken and vegetable soup hot.

The key fertility-supporting ingredients in this recipe are:

- Chicken: A lean protein source that provides zinc, which is important for fertility.
- Quinoa: A whole grain that's high in protein, fiber, and B vitamins.
- Kale/spinach: Leafy greens rich in folate, iron, and antioxidants.
- Flaxseed: Provides omega-3s and lignans that can help balance hormones.
- Pumpkin seeds: A good source of zinc, which is crucial for male and female fertility.

This hearty, nutrient-dense soup is a great option for couples trying to conceive. The combination of protein, complex carbs, vegetables, and fertility-boosting seeds makes it a nourishing and delicious meal.

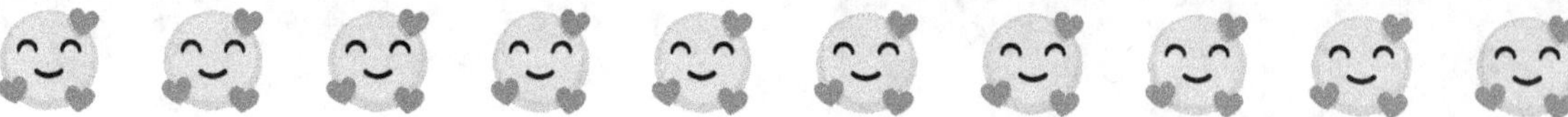

46. Mushroom barley soup with fresh herbs

 Prep Time :   Cook Time :   Servings :

Is this dish easy or difficult for you to make?

 ◯   ◯

Write 5 ....
friends
with   ....
whom
you   ....
want to
share   ....
this
dish   ....

INGREDIENTS

- 1 tbsp olive oil
- 1 onion, diced
- 3 cloves garlic, minced
- 8 oz cremini or button
mushrooms, sliced
- 1 cup pearl barley, rinsed
- 6 cups low-sodium vegetable or
chicken broth
- 2 cups chopped kale or spinach
- 2 tbsp chopped fresh parsley
- 2 tbsp chopped fresh thyme
- Salt and pepper to taste

For Fertility Support:
- 2 tbsp ground flaxseed
- 1 tbsp pumpkin seeds, chopped

How would you rate this dish?

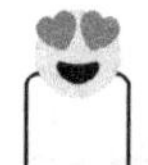 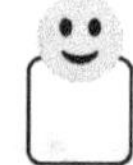  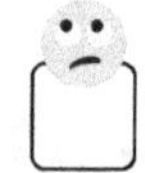 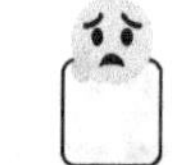

1. In a large pot, heat the olive oil over medium heat. Add the onion and sauté for 5 minutes until translucent.

2. Add the garlic and mushrooms. Sauté for 3-4 minutes until the mushrooms are lightly browned.

3. Stir in the pearl barley and broth. Bring to a boil, then reduce heat and simmer for 25-30 minutes, until the barley is tender.

4. Stir in the kale/spinach, parsley, and thyme. Season with salt and pepper.

5. Remove from heat and stir in the ground flaxseed and chopped pumpkin seeds. Serve the mushroom barley soup hot.

The key fertility-supporting ingredients in this recipe are:

- Mushrooms: Rich in antioxidants and vitamin D, which may improve fertility.

- Barley: A whole grain that's high in fiber, selenium, and B vitamins.

- Kale/spinach: Leafy greens packed with folate, iron, and other fertility-boosting nutrients.

- Flaxseed: Provides omega-3s and lignans that can help balance hormones.

- Pumpkin seeds: A good source of zinc, which is crucial for male and female fertility.

The fresh herbs add flavor and additional antioxidants to this nourishing soup. This hearty, nutrient-dense dish is a great option for couples trying to conceive. The combination of whole grains, vegetables, and fertility-boosting seeds makes it a delicious and healthy meal.

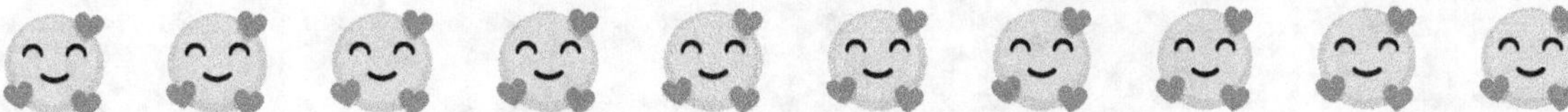

47. Carrot ginger soup with a dollop of Greek yogurt

Let's do that and fill in the time here

 Prep Time :   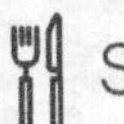 Cook Time :   Servings :

Is this dish easy or difficult for you to make?

◯   ◯

Write 5 friends with whom you want to share this dish ....
....
....
....
....

INGREDIENTS

- 1 tbsp olive oil
- 1 onion, diced
- 3 cloves garlic, minced
- 1 lb carrots, peeled and chopped
- 1 tbsp grated fresh ginger
- 4 cups vegetable or chicken broth
- 1 tsp ground cumin
- Salt and pepper to taste

For Serving:
- 1 cup plain Greek yogurt
- 2 tbsp chopped fresh cilantro

For Fertility Support:
- 1 tbsp ground flaxseed
- 1 tbsp pumpkin seeds, chopped

1. In a large pot, heat the olive oil over medium heat. Add the onion and sauté for 5 minutes until translucent.

2. Add the garlic, carrots, and ginger. Sauté for 3-4 minutes.

3. Pour in the broth and stir in the cumin. Season with salt and pepper.

4. Bring the soup to a boil, then reduce heat and simmer for 20-25 minutes, until the carrots are very soft.

5. Use an immersion blender to puree the soup until smooth.

6. Ladle the carrot ginger soup into bowls. Top each serving with a dollop of Greek yogurt and a sprinkle of chopped cilantro.

7. In a small bowl, mix together the ground flaxseed and chopped pumpkin seeds. Sprinkle this fertility-boosting topping over the soup.

The key fertility-supporting ingredients in this recipe are:

- Carrots: Rich in beta-carotene, an antioxidant that may improve sperm quality.
- Ginger: Contains compounds that may help regulate menstrual cycles and improve fertility.
- Greek yogurt: High in protein, calcium, and probiotics to support reproductive health.
- Flaxseed: Provides omega-3s and lignans that can help balance hormones.
- Pumpkin seeds: A good source of zinc, which is crucial for male and female fertility.

How would you rate this dish?

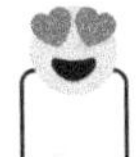 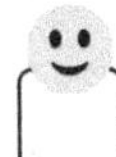  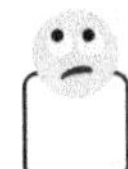 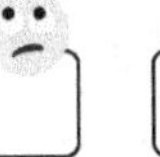 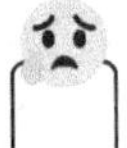

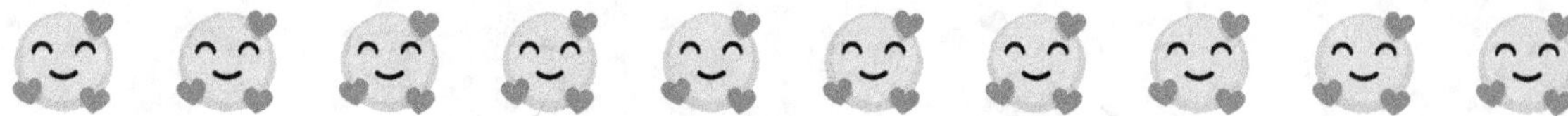

48. Broccoli and cheddar soup (light on cheese)

 Prep Time :    Cook Time :   Servings :

Is this dish easy or difficult for you to make?

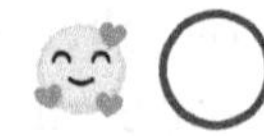 ◯   ◯

Write 5 ....
friends
with   ....
whom
you   ....
want to
share   ....
this
dish   ....

INGREDIENTS

- 1 tbsp olive oil
- 1 onion, diced
- 3 cloves garlic, minced
- 4 cups chopped broccoli florets
- 3 cups low-sodium chicken or vegetable broth
- 1/2 cup shredded low-fat cheddar cheese
- 1/4 cup plain Greek yogurt
- 1 tsp Dijon mustard
- Salt and pepper to taste

For Fertility Support:
- 2 tbsp ground flaxseed
- 1 tbsp chopped walnuts

How would you rate this dish?

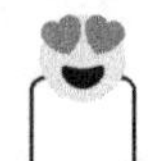 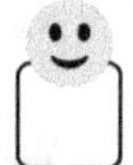 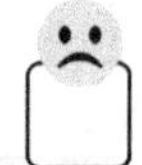 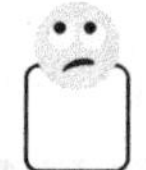 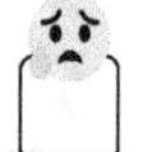

1. In a large pot, heat the olive oil over medium heat. Add the onion and sauté for 5 minutes until translucent.

2. Add the garlic and broccoli. Sauté for 3-4 minutes.

3. Pour in the broth and bring to a boil. Reduce heat and simmer for 15-20 minutes, until the broccoli is very tender.

4. Use an immersion blender to puree the soup until smooth.

5. Stir in the cheddar cheese, Greek yogurt, and Dijon mustard. Season with salt and pepper.

6. Remove from heat and stir in the ground flaxseed and chopped walnuts. Serve the broccoli cheddar soup warm.

The key fertility-supporting ingredients in this recipe are:

- Broccoli: Rich in antioxidants, folate, and fiber to support reproductive health.
- Greek yogurt: High in protein, calcium, and probiotics.
- Flaxseed: Provides omega-3s and lignans that can help balance hormones.
- Walnuts: A good source of omega-3s, zinc, and folate - all important for fertility.

By using a lighter hand with the cheese and adding in fertility-boosting ingredients like flaxseed and walnuts, this broccoli cheddar soup becomes a nourishing and delicious option for couples trying to conceive. The creaminess from the Greek yogurt helps balance the flavors without needing as much cheese.

Enjoy this comforting, nutrient-dense soup as a light meal or appetizer.

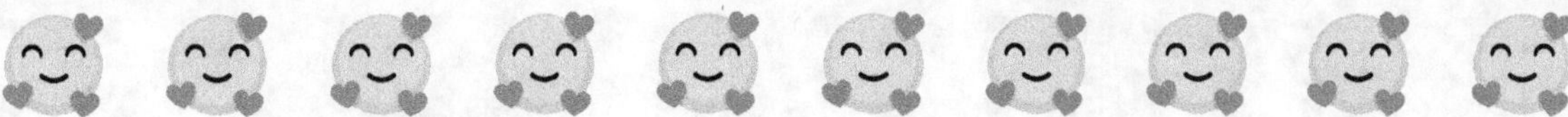

49. Sweet potato and black bean soup with cumin

Prep Time :  Cook Time :  Servings :

Is this dish easy or difficult for you to make?

Write 5 friends with whom you want to share this dish

....

....

....

....

....

INGREDIENTS

- 1 tbsp olive oil
- 1 onion, diced
- 3 cloves garlic, minced
- 2 medium sweet potatoes, peeled and cubed
- 1 (15 oz) can black beans, rinsed and drained
- 4 cups low-sodium vegetable or chicken broth
- 1 tsp ground cumin
- 1 tsp chili powder
- Salt and pepper to taste

For Fertility Support:
- 2 tbsp ground flaxseed
- 1 tbsp pumpkin seeds, chopped

1. In a large pot, heat the olive oil over medium heat. Add the onion and sauté for 5 minutes until translucent.

2. Add the garlic and sauté for 1 minute until fragrant.

3. Stir in the cubed sweet potatoes, black beans, broth, cumin, and chili powder. Season with salt and pepper.

4. Bring the soup to a boil, then reduce heat and simmer for 20-25 minutes, until the sweet potatoes are very soft.

5. Use an immersion blender to partially puree the soup, leaving some texture.

6. Remove from heat and stir in the ground flaxseed and chopped pumpkin seeds.

7. Serve the sweet potato and black bean soup hot.

The key fertility-supporting ingredients in this recipe are:

- Sweet potatoes: Rich in beta-carotene, an antioxidant that may improve sperm quality and female fertility.
- Black beans: High in protein, fiber, and folate to support reproductive health.
- Cumin: Contains compounds that may help regulate menstrual cycles and improve fertility.
- Flaxseed: Provides omega-3s and lignans that can help balance hormones.
- Pumpkin seeds: A good source of zinc, which is crucial for male and female fertility.

This hearty, nutrient-dense soup makes a delicious and nourishing meal for couples trying to conceive. The combination of sweet potatoes, black beans, warming spices, and fertility-boosting seeds provides a satisfying and fertility-supporting dish.

How would you rate this dish?

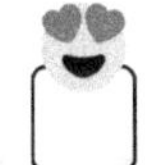 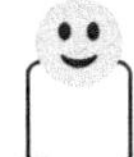  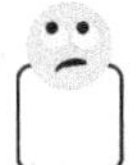 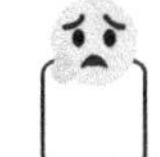

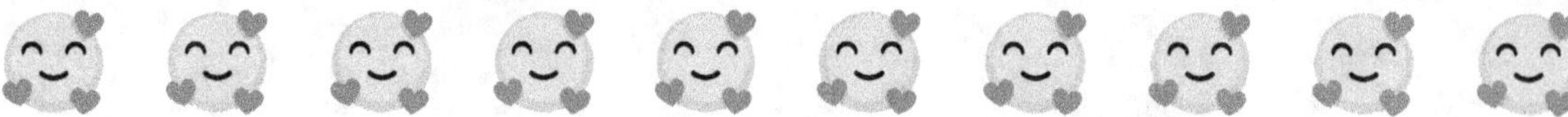

50. Red lentil soup with lemon and spinach

Prep Time :   Cook Time :   Servings :

Is this dish easy or difficult for you to make?

 ◯    ◯

Write 5 ....
friends
with ....
whom
you ....
want to
share ....
this
dish ....

INGREDIENTS

- 1 tbsp olive oil
- 1 onion, diced
- 3 cloves garlic, minced
- 1 cup red lentils, rinsed
- 6 cups low-sodium vegetable or chicken broth
- 1 tsp ground cumin
- 1 tsp ground coriander
- Juice of 1 lemon
- 2 cups chopped fresh spinach
- Salt and pepper to taste

1. In a large pot, heat the olive oil over medium heat. Add the onion and sauté for 5 minutes until translucent.

2. Add the garlic and sauté for 1 minute until fragrant.

3. Stir in the rinsed red lentils, broth, cumin, and coriander. Season with salt and pepper.

4. Bring the soup to a boil, then reduce heat and simmer for 20-25 minutes, until the lentils are very soft.

5. Remove from heat and stir in the lemon juice and chopped spinach. Allow the spinach to wilt for 1-2 minutes. Serve the red lentil soup hot.

This red lentil soup is packed with nutrients that support overall health, including:

- Red lentils: An excellent source of plant-based protein, fiber, and folate.
- Spinach: Rich in vitamins A, C, and K, as well as iron and antioxidants.
- Lemon: Provides vitamin C and can help enhance iron absorption.
- Cumin and coriander: Warming spices that add flavor and may have anti-inflammatory properties.

The combination of protein-rich lentils, nutrient-dense spinach, and the bright, tangy flavor of lemon makes this a nourishing and delicious soup. It's a great option for a light meal or starter.

Enjoy this red lentil soup as part of a balanced, healthy diet. The wholesome ingredients provide a boost of essential vitamins and minerals to support overall wellness.

How would you rate this dish?

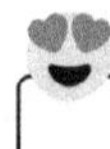 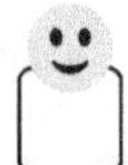 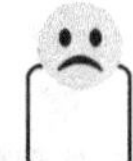 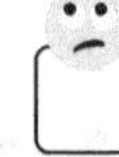 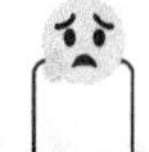

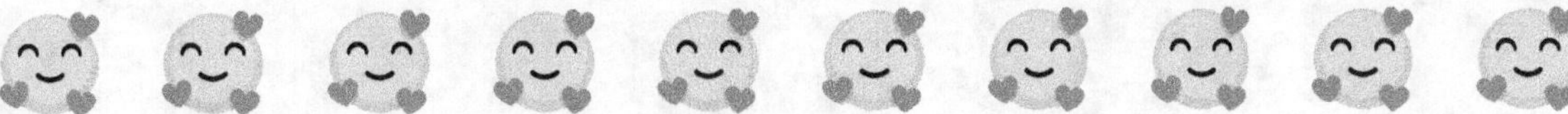

51. Kale and quinoa salad with cranberries and almonds

 Prep Time :   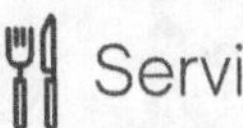 Cook Time :   Servings :

Is this dish easy or difficult for you to make?

◯   ◯

Write 5 friends with whom you want to share this dish

....
....
....
....
....

INGREDIENTS

- 1 cup cooked quinoa, cooled
- 4 cups chopped kale, stems removed
- 1/2 cup dried cranberries
- 1/4 cup sliced almonds
- 2 tbsp olive oil
- 2 tbsp apple cider vinegar
- 1 tbsp Dijon mustard
- 1 tbsp honey
- Salt and pepper to taste

For Fertility Support:
- 2 tbsp ground flaxseed
- 1 tbsp pumpkin seeds, chopped

1. In a large bowl, combine the cooked quinoa, chopped kale, dried cranberries, and sliced almonds.

2. In a small bowl, whisk together the olive oil, apple cider vinegar, Dijon mustard, and honey. Season with salt and pepper.

3. Pour the dressing over the kale and quinoa mixture and toss to coat evenly.

4. Sprinkle the ground flaxseed and chopped pumpkin seeds over the top of the salad.

5. Serve the kale and quinoa salad immediately or refrigerate until ready to serve.

The key fertility-supporting ingredients in this recipe are:

- Kale: A nutrient-dense leafy green that's high in folate, iron, and antioxidants.
- Quinoa: A complete protein source that's also high in fiber and B vitamins.
- Cranberries: Rich in antioxidants that may help improve fertility.
- Almonds: A good source of healthy fats, protein, and vitamins important for reproductive health.
- Flaxseed: Provides omega-3s and lignans that can help balance hormones.
- Pumpkin seeds: High in zinc, which is crucial for male and female fertility.

This colorful, nutrient-packed salad makes a delicious and fertility-boosting meal or side dish. The combination of superfoods like kale, quinoa, and nuts/seeds provides a nourishing boost of vitamins, minerals, and antioxidants to support overall reproductive health.

How would you rate this dish?

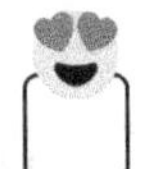 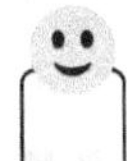  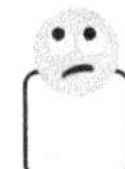 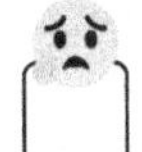

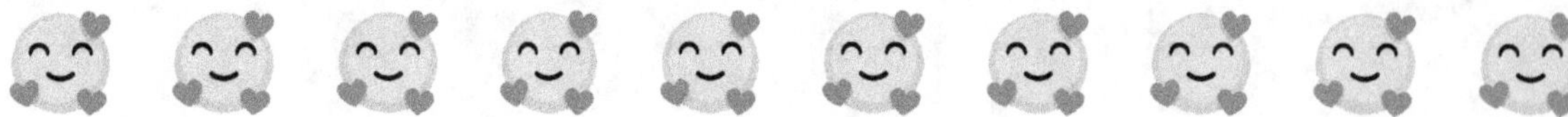

52. Spinach and avocado salad with sunflower seeds

 Prep Time :   Cook Time :   Servings :

Is this dish easy or difficult for you to make?

○   ○

Write 5 friends with whom you want to share this dish ....

....

....

....

....

INGREDIENTS

- 5 cups fresh spinach, washed and chopped
- 1 avocado, diced
- 1/4 cup sunflower seeds
- 2 tbsp olive oil
- 1 tbsp apple cider vinegar
- 1 tsp Dijon mustard
- 1 tsp honey
- Salt and pepper to taste

For Fertility Support:
- 1 tbsp ground flaxseed
- 1 tbsp chopped walnuts

1. In a large salad bowl, combine the chopped spinach, diced avocado, and sunflower seeds.

2. In a small bowl, whisk together the olive oil, apple cider vinegar, Dijon mustard, and honey. Season with salt and pepper.

3. Pour the dressing over the spinach and avocado salad and toss gently to coat.

4. Sprinkle the ground flaxseed and chopped walnuts over the top of the salad.

5. Serve the spinach and avocado salad immediately.

The key fertility-supporting ingredients in this recipe are:

- Spinach: A nutrient-dense leafy green that's high in folate, iron, and antioxidants.
- Avocado: Rich in healthy fats, vitamins, and antioxidants that support reproductive health.
- Sunflower seeds: A good source of zinc, which is crucial for male and female fertility.
- Flaxseed: Provides omega-3s and lignans that can help balance hormones.
- Walnuts: High in omega-3s, zinc, and folate - all important for fertility.

This simple, nourishing salad provides a delicious way to incorporate fertility-boosting ingredients into your diet. The combination of leafy greens, healthy fats, and nutrient-dense seeds and nuts makes it a great option for couples trying to conceive.

Enjoy this spinach and avocado salad as a light meal or side dish.

How would you rate this dish?

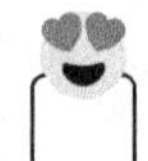 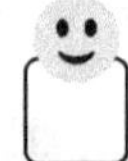 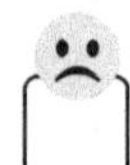 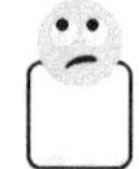 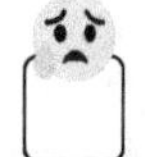

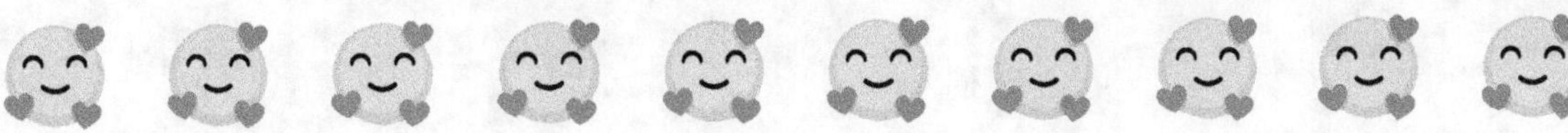

53. Arugula and beet salad with goat cheese

Prep Time :   Cook Time :   Servings :

Is this dish easy or difficult for you to make?

 ◯   😊 ◯

Write 5 friends with whom you want to share this dish

....
....
....
....
....

INGREDIENTS

- 5 cups arugula, washed and chopped
- 2 medium beets, roasted, peeled, and sliced
- 1/4 cup crumbled goat cheese
- 2 tbsp olive oil
- 1 tbsp balsamic vinegar
- 1 tsp Dijon mustard
- Salt and pepper to taste

For Fertility Support:
- 2 tbsp ground flaxseed
- 1 tbsp chopped walnuts

1. In a large salad bowl, combine the chopped arugula, roasted beet slices, and crumbled goat cheese.

2. In a small bowl, whisk together the olive oil, balsamic vinegar, and Dijon mustard. Season with salt and pepper.

3. Drizzle the dressing over the arugula and beet salad, then toss gently to coat.

4. Sprinkle the ground flaxseed and chopped walnuts over the top of the salad.

5. Serve the arugula and beet salad immediately.

The key fertility-supporting ingredients in this recipe are:

- Arugula: A nutrient-dense leafy green that's high in folate, calcium, and antioxidants.
- Beets: Rich in betalains, an antioxidant that may improve sperm quality and female fertility.
- Goat cheese: A source of protein and calcium to support reproductive health.
- Flaxseed: Provides omega-3s and lignans that can help balance hormones.
- Walnuts: High in omega-3s, zinc, and folate - all important for fertility.

This colorful, nutrient-packed salad makes a delicious and fertility-boosting meal or side dish. The combination of peppery arugula, sweet roasted beets, creamy goat cheese, and the added benefits of flaxseed and walnuts provide a nourishing boost of vitamins, minerals, and antioxidants to support overall reproductive health.

How would you rate this dish?

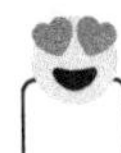  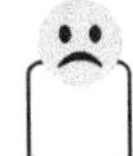 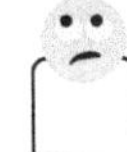 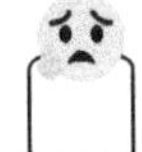

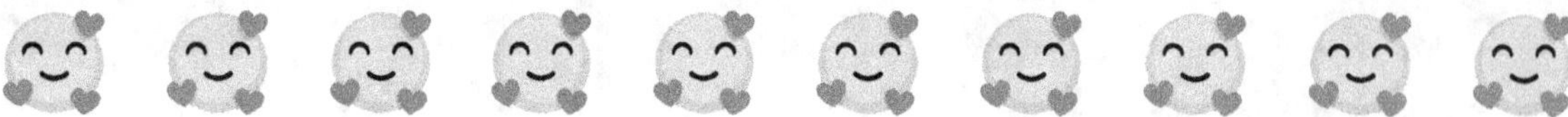

54. Chickpea and cucumber salad with dill dressing

 Prep Time :   Cook Time :   Servings :

Is this dish easy or difficult for you to make?

 ◯   ◯

Write 5 ....
friends
with ....
whom
you ....
want to
share ....
this
dish ....

INGREDIENTS

- 1 (15 oz) can chickpeas, drained and rinsed
- 1 cucumber, diced
- 1/2 red onion, thinly sliced
- 1/4 cup fresh dill, chopped
- 2 tbsp olive oil
- 2 tbsp white wine vinegar
- 1 tbsp Dijon mustard
- 1 tsp honey
- Salt and pepper to taste

1. In a large bowl, combine the chickpeas, cucumber, red onion, and fresh dill.

2. In a small bowl, whisk together the olive oil, white wine vinegar, Dijon mustard, and honey. Season with salt and pepper.

3. Pour the dressing over the chickpea and cucumber mixture and toss gently to coat.

4. Refrigerate for at least 30 minutes to allow the flavors to meld.

5. Serve chilled or at room temperature. Enjoy!

The dill dressing adds a bright, herbal flavor that pairs perfectly with the chickpeas and crisp cucumber. This salad makes a great side dish or light main course. Feel free to adjust the amounts of any ingredients to suit your taste preferences.

How would you rate this dish?

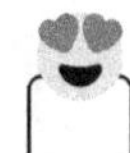 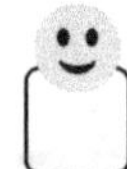 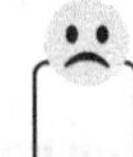 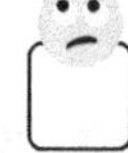 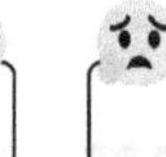

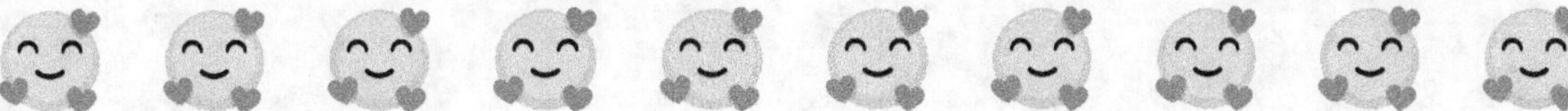

55. Mediterranean salad with olives, cucumber, and feta

 Prep Time :   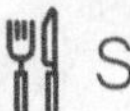 Cook Time :   Servings :

Is this dish easy or difficult for you to make?

○   ○

Write 5 ....
friends
with   ....
whom
you   ....
want to
share   ....
this
dish   ....

INGREDIENTS

- 1 cucumber, diced
- 1 cup cherry tomatoes, halved
- 1/2 red onion, thinly sliced
- 1 cup Kalamata olives, pitted and halved
- 1 cup crumbled feta cheese
- 1/4 cup fresh parsley, chopped
- 2 tbsp olive oil
- 2 tbsp red wine vinegar
- 1 tsp dried oregano
- Salt and pepper to taste

How would you rate this dish?

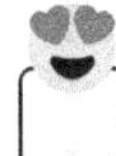 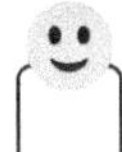  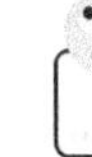 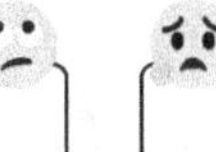

1. In a large bowl, combine the diced cucumber, cherry tomatoes, red onion, Kalamata olives, crumbled feta, and chopped parsley.

2. In a small bowl, whisk together the olive oil, red wine vinegar, and dried oregano. Season with salt and pepper.

3. Pour the dressing over the salad and toss gently to coat.

4. Refrigerate for at least 30 minutes to allow the flavors to meld.

5. Serve chilled or at room temperature.

This Mediterranean-inspired salad is packed with fertility-supporting nutrients:

- Cucumbers are a good source of silica, which can help improve sperm motility.

- Olives and olive oil contain healthy fats that can support hormone balance.

- Feta cheese is a good source of zinc, which is important for male fertility.

- Tomatoes contain lycopene, an antioxidant that may help protect sperm.

- Parsley is a natural diuretic and can help flush out toxins.

The combination of fresh vegetables, healthy fats, and antioxidants makes this salad a great choice for couples trying to conceive. Enjoy!

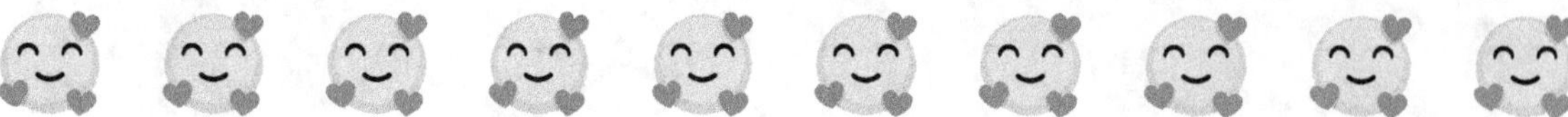

56. Roasted vegetable salad with balsamic glaze

Prep Time :   Cook Time :   Servings :

Is this dish easy or difficult for you to make?

 ◯    ◯

Write 5 friends with whom you want to share this dish

....

....

....

....

....

INGREDIENTS

- 1 medium zucchini, sliced into 1/2-inch rounds
- 1 red bell pepper, cut into 1-inch pieces
- 1 yellow bell pepper, cut into 1-inch pieces
- 1 red onion, cut into 1-inch wedges
- 8 oz cremini mushrooms, halved
- 2 tbsp olive oil
- Salt and pepper to taste
- 5 oz mixed greens
- 1/4 cup crumbled feta cheese
- 2 tbsp balsamic glaze

1. Preheat oven to 400°F. Line a large baking sheet with parchment paper.

2. In a large bowl, toss the zucchini, bell peppers, red onion, and mushrooms with the olive oil. Season with salt and pepper.

3. Spread the vegetables in a single layer on the prepared baking sheet. Roast for 20-25 minutes, stirring halfway, until vegetables are tender and lightly browned.

4. Allow the roasted vegetables to cool slightly.

5. In a large salad bowl, combine the mixed greens, roasted vegetables, and crumbled feta cheese.

6. Drizzle the balsamic glaze over the top of the salad and toss gently to coat.

7. Serve immediately.

The roasted vegetables add a delicious depth of flavor to this salad, while the balsamic glaze provides a sweet and tangy finish. The feta cheese adds a creamy, salty element. This salad makes a great main dish or side. Enjoy!

How would you rate this dish?

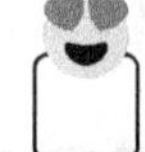 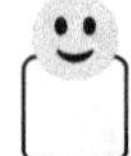 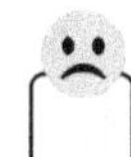 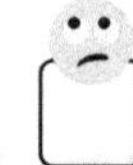 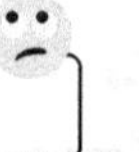 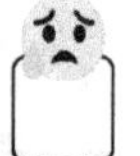

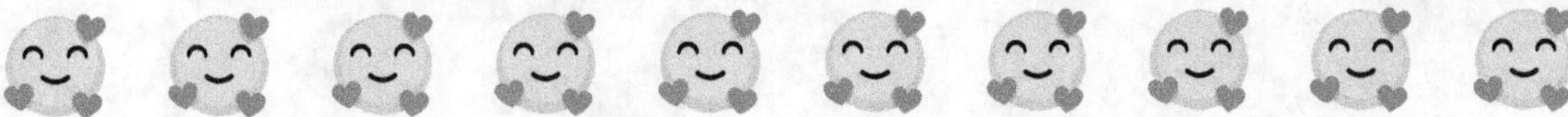

Let's do that and fill in the time here

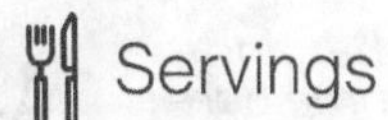 Prep Time :   Cook Time :   Servings :

Is this dish easy or difficult for you to make?

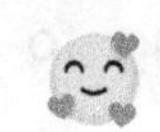 ◯   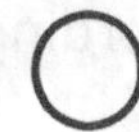 ◯

Write 5 friends with whom you want to share this dish

....

....

....

....

....

INGREDIENTS

- 2 crisp apples, diced (such as Honeycrisp or Gala)
- 1 cup diced celery
- 1/2 cup chopped walnuts
- 1/4 cup mayonnaise
- 2 tbsp plain Greek yogurt
- 1 tbsp lemon juice
- 1 tsp honey
- Salt and pepper to taste
- Lettuce leaves for serving (optional)

1. In a large bowl, combine the diced apples, celery, and chopped walnuts.

2. In a small bowl, whisk together the mayonnaise, Greek yogurt, lemon juice, and honey. Season with salt and pepper.

3. Pour the dressing over the apple, celery, and walnut mixture and toss gently to coat.

4. Cover and refrigerate for at least 30 minutes to allow the flavors to meld.

5. Serve the Waldorf salad on a bed of lettuce leaves, if desired.

The classic combination of crisp apples, crunchy celery, and toasted walnuts makes this Waldorf salad a delicious and refreshing side dish or light main course. The creamy dressing ties all the flavors together.

Some variations you could try:
- Add grapes, raisins, or dried cranberries
- Use plain yogurt instead of Greek yogurt
- Sprinkle with a bit of chopped parsley or chives

Enjoy this timeless Waldorf salad!

How would you rate this dish?

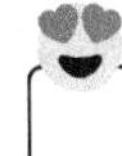 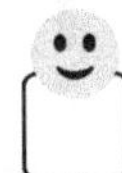  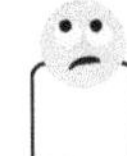 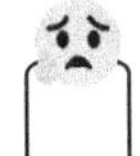

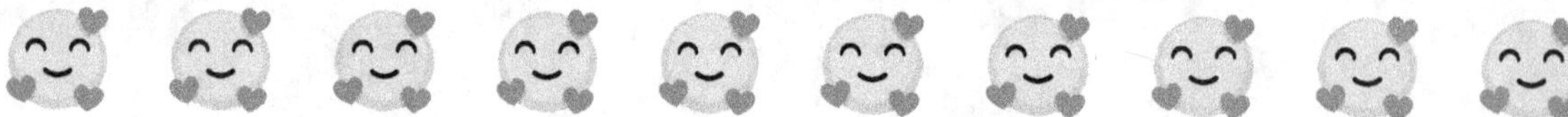

58. Farro salad with cherry tomatoes and basil

Prep Time :   Cook Time :   Servings :

Is this dish easy or difficult for you to make?

 ○   ○

Write 5 friends with whom you want to share this dish

....
....
....
....
....

INGREDIENTS

- 1 cup uncooked farro
- 1 pint cherry tomatoes, halved
- 1 cup fresh basil leaves, chopped
- 1/2 red onion, thinly sliced
- 2 tbsp olive oil
- 2 tbsp balsamic vinegar
- 1 tsp Dijon mustard
- 1 tsp honey
- Salt and pepper to taste

1. Cook the farro according to package instructions. Drain and let cool.

2. In a large bowl, combine the cooked farro, cherry tomatoes, chopped basil, and sliced red onion.

3. In a small bowl, whisk together the olive oil, balsamic vinegar, Dijon mustard, and honey. Season with salt and pepper.

4. Pour the dressing over the farro salad and toss gently to coat.

5. Refrigerate for at least 30 minutes to allow the flavors to meld. Serve chilled or at room temperature.

This farro salad is packed with fertility-supporting nutrients:

- Farro is a whole grain that's high in fiber, protein, and antioxidants.
- Cherry tomatoes contain lycopene, an antioxidant that may help protect sperm.
- Basil is a natural anti-inflammatory and can help improve blood flow.
- Olive oil and balsamic vinegar provide healthy fats that support hormone balance.

The combination of whole grains, vegetables, and healthy fats makes this salad a great choice for couples trying to conceive. It can be enjoyed as a main dish or a side.

Feel free to adjust the amounts of any ingredients to suit your taste preferences. Enjoy!

How would you rate this dish?

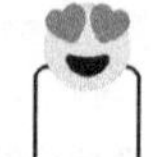 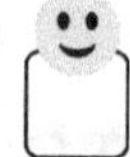 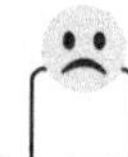 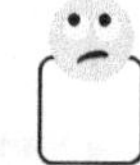 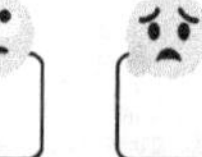

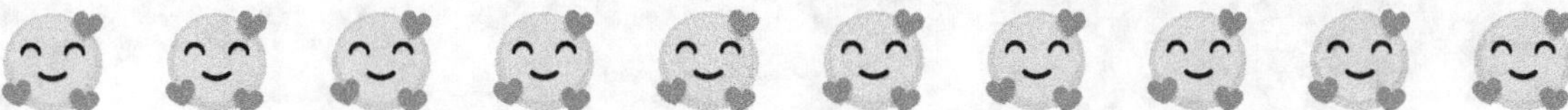

59. Orzo salad with grilled zucchini and feta

 Prep Time :    Cook Time :   Servings :

Is this dish easy or difficult for you to make?

Write 5 friends with whom you want to share this dish ....

INGREDIENTS

- 1 cup uncooked orzo pasta
- 2 medium zucchini, sliced into 1/2-inch rounds
- 2 tbsp olive oil, divided
- 1 cup crumbled feta cheese
- 1/2 cup cherry tomatoes, halved
- 1/4 cup chopped fresh basil
- 2 tbsp lemon juice
- 1 tsp Dijon mustard
- Salt and pepper to taste

How would you rate this dish?

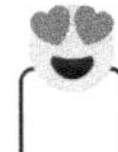  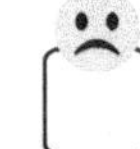 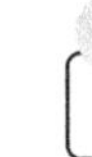 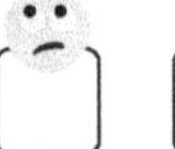 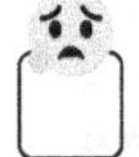

1. Cook the orzo according to package instructions. Drain and rinse with cold water.

2. Preheat grill or grill pan to medium-high heat. Brush the zucchini slices with 1 tbsp of the olive oil and season with salt and pepper.

3. Grill the zucchini for 2-3 minutes per side, until tender and lightly charred. Remove from heat and let cool slightly, then chop into bite-sized pieces.

4. In a large bowl, combine the cooked orzo, grilled zucchini, feta cheese, cherry tomatoes, and chopped basil.

5. In a small bowl, whisk together the remaining 1 tbsp olive oil, lemon juice, and Dijon mustard. Season with salt and pepper.

6. Pour the dressing over the orzo salad and toss gently to coat.

7. Refrigerate for at least 30 minutes to allow the flavors to meld. Serve chilled or at room temperature.

This orzo salad is packed with fertility-supporting ingredients:

- Orzo is a type of pasta made from wheat, providing complex carbs and fiber.
- Zucchini is a good source of antioxidants like vitamin C and zinc.
- Feta cheese is high in protein and zinc, which are important for male fertility.
- Tomatoes contain lycopene, an antioxidant that may help protect sperm.
- Basil and olive oil provide anti-inflammatory benefits.

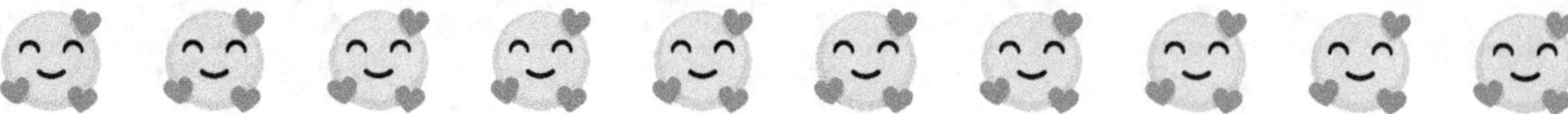

60. Mixed greens with mandarin oranges and almonds

 Prep Time :    Cook Time :   Servings :

Is this dish easy or difficult for you to make?

⊗ ◯   ☺ ◯

Write 5 friends with whom you want to share this dish

....
....
....
....
....

INGREDIENTS

- 5 oz mixed greens (such as spinach, arugula, and kale)
- 1 (11 oz) can mandarin oranges, drained
- 1/4 cup sliced almonds, toasted
- 2 tbsp olive oil
- 1 tbsp balsamic vinegar
- 1 tsp Dijon mustard
- 1 tsp honey
- Salt and pepper to taste

1. In a large salad bowl, combine the mixed greens, mandarin oranges, and toasted almond slices.

2. In a small bowl, whisk together the olive oil, balsamic vinegar, Dijon mustard, and honey. Season with salt and pepper.

3. Drizzle the dressing over the salad and toss gently to coat. Serve immediately.

This salad is packed with fertility-supporting nutrients:

- Mixed greens like spinach and kale are rich in folate, which is important for both male and female fertility.

- Mandarin oranges are a good source of vitamin C, an antioxidant that can help protect sperm.

- Almonds contain healthy fats, protein, and antioxidants like vitamin E that may improve sperm quality.

- Olive oil and balsamic vinegar provide anti-inflammatory benefits.

The combination of nutrient-dense greens, citrus, and nuts makes this salad a great choice for couples trying to conceive. The bright, tangy dressing complements the sweetness of the mandarin oranges.

Feel free to adjust the amounts of any ingredients to suit your taste preferences. Enjoy this fertility-boosting salad!

How would you rate this dish?

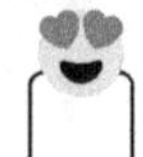 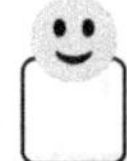 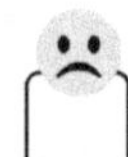 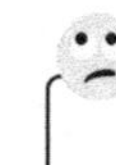 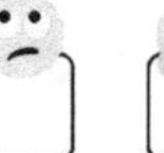 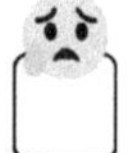

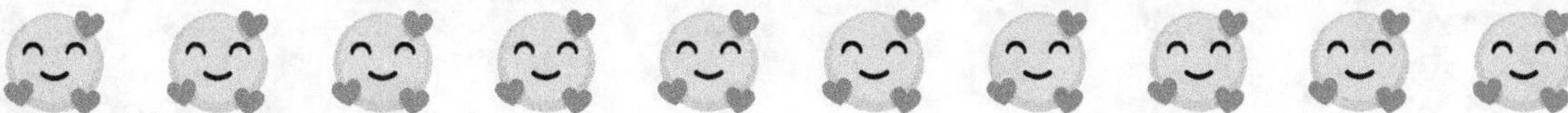

61. Stuffed zucchini boats with quinoa and vegetables

Prep Time :   Cook Time :   Servings :

Is this dish easy or difficult for you to make?

 ◯    ◯

Write 5 friends with whom you want to share this dish ....

INGREDIENTS

- 4 medium zucchini, halved lengthwise
- 1 cup cooked quinoa
- 1/2 cup diced bell pepper
- 1/2 cup diced onion
- 1 cup diced mushrooms
- 2 cloves garlic, minced
- 1/4 cup crumbled feta cheese
- 2 tbsp chopped fresh parsley
- 2 tbsp olive oil
- Salt and pepper to taste

1. Preheat oven to 375°F. Scoop out the flesh from the zucchini halves, leaving a 1/4-inch shell. Finely chop the zucchini flesh.

2. In a skillet, heat the olive oil over medium heat. Add the chopped zucchini flesh, bell pepper, onion, mushrooms, and garlic. Sauté for 5-7 minutes until vegetables are tender.

3. Remove the skillet from heat and stir in the cooked quinoa, feta cheese, and parsley. Season with salt and pepper.

4. Spoon the quinoa mixture evenly into the zucchini boats.

5. Place the stuffed zucchini boats on a baking sheet and bake for 20-25 minutes, until the zucchini is tender.

6. Serve warm.

This stuffed zucchini dish is packed with fertility-supporting nutrients:

- Zucchini is a good source of antioxidants like vitamin C and zinc.
- Quinoa is a whole grain that's high in protein, fiber, and B vitamins.
- Bell peppers contain vitamin C, which can help improve sperm quality.
- Mushrooms are a source of selenium, an important mineral for male fertility.
- Feta cheese provides protein and zinc.
- Olive oil and parsley offer anti-inflammatory benefits.

The combination of vegetables, whole grains, and healthy fats makes this a great meal for couples trying to conceive. Adjust the vegetable fillings to your liking. Enjoy!

How would you rate this dish?

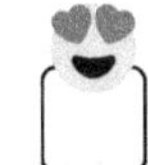 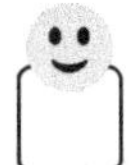  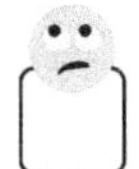 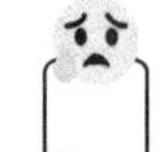

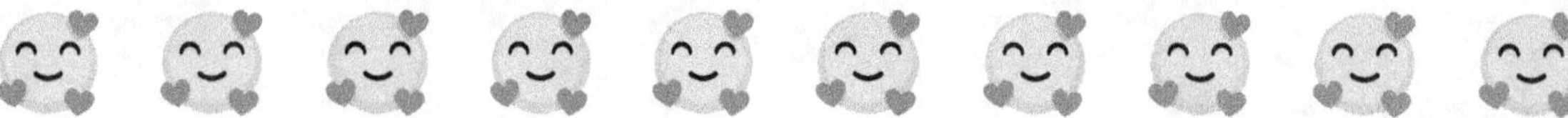

62. Black bean and corn tacos with avocado

Let's do that and fill in the time here ✓ Prep Time :   🕐 Cook Time :   🍴 Servings :

Is this dish easy or difficult for you to make?

 ◯   🙂 ◯

Write 5 friends with whom you want to share this dish
....
....
....
....
....

INGREDIENTS

- 1 (15 oz) can black beans, drained and rinsed
- 1 cup frozen corn kernels, thawed
- 1 tsp cumin
- 1 tsp chili powder
- Salt and pepper to taste
- 8-10 small corn tortillas
- 1 avocado, diced
- 1/4 cup crumbled queso fresco or feta cheese
- 2 tbsp chopped cilantro
- Lime wedges for serving

How would you rate this dish?

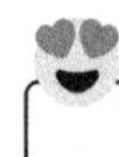 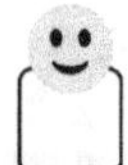 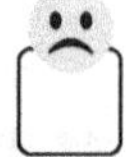 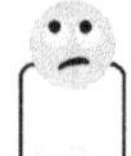 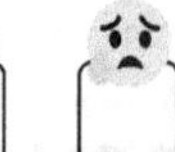

1. In a medium saucepan, combine the black beans, corn, cumin, chili powder, and a pinch of salt and pepper. Cook over medium heat, stirring occasionally, until heated through, about 5 minutes.

2. Warm the corn tortillas according to package instructions.

3. To assemble the tacos, place a spoonful of the black bean and corn mixture into each tortilla. Top with diced avocado, crumbled queso fresco or feta, and chopped cilantro.

4. Serve the tacos with lime wedges on the side.

This taco recipe is packed with fertility-supporting ingredients:

- Black beans are a great source of folate, zinc, and protein.

- Corn contains antioxidants like lutein and zeaxanthin that may help protect sperm.

- Avocado is rich in healthy fats, vitamin E, and folate, all important for fertility.

- Queso fresco or feta cheese provides protein and zinc.

- Cilantro is a natural diuretic and can help flush out toxins.

The combination of fiber-rich beans, antioxidant-packed vegetables, and healthy fats makes this a nutritious and delicious meal for couples trying to conceive. Feel free to adjust the spices or toppings to your taste preferences. Enjoy!

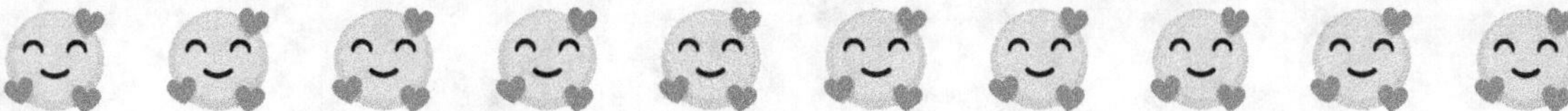

63. Spaghetti squash with marinara sauce

Prep Time :   Cook Time :   Servings :

Is this dish easy or difficult for you to make?

 ◯    ◯

Write 5 friends with whom you want to share this dish

....

....

....

....

....

INGREDIENTS

- 1 medium spaghetti squash, halved lengthwise and seeds removed
- 2 tbsp olive oil
- Salt and pepper to taste
- 1 (24 oz) jar marinara sauce
- 1/4 cup grated Parmesan cheese (optional)
- 2 tbsp chopped fresh basil (optional)

How would you rate this dish?

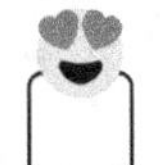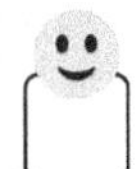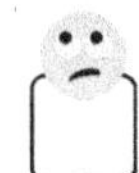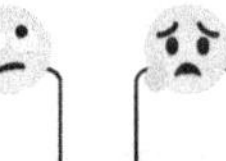

1. Preheat oven to 400°F. Line a baking sheet with parchment paper.

2. Place the spaghetti squash halves cut-side up on the prepared baking sheet. Drizzle with olive oil and season with salt and pepper.

3. Roast the spaghetti squash for 40-50 minutes, until tender when pierced with a fork.

4. Remove the spaghetti squash from the oven and let cool slightly. Using a fork, gently scrape the flesh into strands.

5. In a large skillet, heat the marinara sauce over medium heat until warmed through.

6. Add the spaghetti squash strands to the marinara sauce and toss to coat.

7. Serve the spaghetti squash with marinara sauce, topped with grated Parmesan cheese and chopped fresh basil, if desired.

This spaghetti squash dish is a great fertility-supporting meal:

- Spaghetti squash is a nutrient-dense vegetable that's high in folate, vitamin C, and antioxidants.
- Marinara sauce is a good source of lycopene, an antioxidant that may help protect sperm.
- Parmesan cheese provides protein and zinc, which are important for male fertility.
- Basil is a natural anti-inflammatory and can help improve blood flow.

The combination of the nutrient-rich spaghetti squash, antioxidant-packed marinara sauce, and fertility-boosting toppings makes this a great choice for couples trying to conceive. Enjoy!

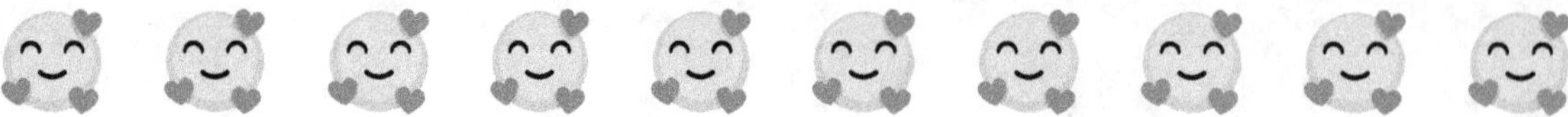

64. Vegetable stir-fry with tofu and brown rice

Let's do that and fill in the time here

Prep Time :

Cook Time :

Servings :

Is this dish easy or difficult for you to make?

 ○   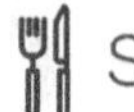 ○

Write 5 friends with whom you want to share this dish

....
....
....
....
....

INGREDIENTS

- 1 cup uncooked brown rice
- 1 block (14 oz) extra-firm tofu, cubed
- 2 tbsp sesame oil, divided
- 2 cups mixed vegetables (such as broccoli, bell peppers, snow peas, and mushrooms), chopped
- 2 cloves garlic, minced
- 1 tbsp grated fresh ginger
- 2 tbsp low-sodium soy sauce or tamari
- 1 tbsp rice vinegar
- 1 tsp honey
- Salt and pepper to taste
- Chopped green onions and sesame seeds for garnish (optional)

How would you rate this dish?

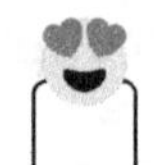 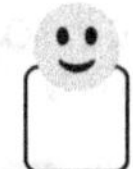 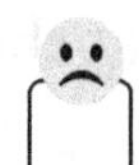 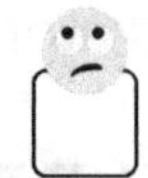 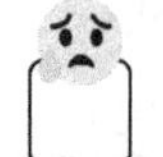

1. Cook the brown rice according to package instructions.

2. In a large skillet or wok, heat 1 tbsp of the sesame oil over medium-high heat. Add the cubed tofu and cook, stirring occasionally, until lightly browned on all sides, about 5-7 minutes. Transfer the tofu to a plate.

3. Add the remaining 1 tbsp of sesame oil to the skillet. Add the chopped vegetables, garlic, and ginger. Stir-fry for 5-7 minutes, until the vegetables are tender-crisp.

4. Return the cooked tofu to the skillet. Add the soy sauce, rice vinegar, and honey. Toss to coat everything evenly.

5. Serve the stir-fry over the cooked brown rice. Garnish with chopped green onions and sesame seeds, if desired.

This vegetable stir-fry is packed with fertility-supporting nutrients:

- Brown rice is a whole grain that's high in fiber, B vitamins, and antioxidants.
- Tofu is a good source of plant-based protein and isoflavones, which may help improve sperm quality.
- Vegetables like broccoli, bell peppers, and mushrooms are rich in antioxidants, vitamins, and minerals that support fertility.
- Ginger and garlic have anti-inflammatory properties that can help improve blood flow.
- Sesame oil and sesame seeds contain healthy fats and nutrients like zinc and selenium.

The combination of nutrient-dense vegetables, protein-rich tofu, and whole grains makes this stir-fry a great choice for couples trying to conceive. Adjust the vegetables to your liking. Enjoy!

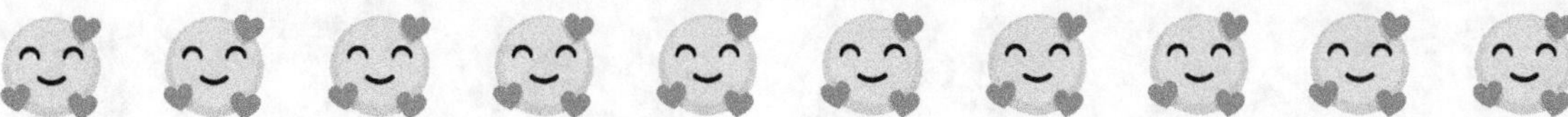

65. Lentil shepherd's pie with mashed sweet potatoes

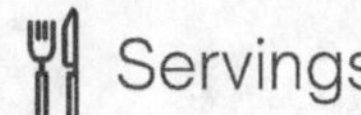 Prep Time :   Cook Time :   Servings :

Is this dish easy or difficult for you to make?

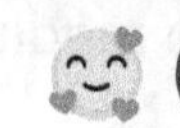 ◯   ◯

Write 5 ....
friends
with ....
whom
you ....
want to
share ....
this
dish ....

INGREDIENTS

For the Filling:
- 1 cup dry brown or green lentils, rinsed
- 3 cups vegetable broth
- 1 tbsp olive oil
- 1 onion, diced
- 3 carrots, peeled and diced
- 3 celery stalks, diced
- 3 cloves garlic, minced
- 1 tsp dried thyme
- 1 tsp dried rosemary
- 1 tsp Worcestershire sauce (use vegan if desired)
- Salt and pepper to taste

For the Topping:
- 3 medium sweet potatoes, peeled and cubed
- 2 tbsp unsweetened almond milk
- 2 tbsp olive oil
- Salt and pepper to taste

1. Preheat oven to 375°F.

2. In a medium saucepan, combine the lentils and vegetable broth. Bring to a boil, then reduce heat and simmer for 20-25 minutes, until lentils are tender. Drain any excess liquid.

3. In a large skillet, heat the 1 tbsp olive oil over medium heat. Add the onion, carrots, celery, and garlic. Sauté for 5-7 minutes, until vegetables are softened.

4. Stir the cooked lentils, thyme, rosemary, Worcestershire sauce, salt, and pepper into the vegetable mixture. Cook for 2-3 minutes more.

5. Transfer the lentil filling to a 9x13 inch baking dish.

6. In a medium pot, cover the sweet potato cubes with water. Bring to a boil and cook until tender, about 15 minutes. Drain and return to the pot.

7. Mash the sweet potatoes with the almond milk and 2 tbsp olive oil. Season with salt and pepper.

8. Spread the mashed sweet potatoes evenly over the lentil filling.

9. Bake for 25-30 minutes, until the sweet potato topping is lightly browned.

10. Let cool for 5-10 minutes before serving.

This hearty lentil shepherd's pie is a delicious vegetarian main dish. The sweet potato topping adds a creamy, comforting element. Enjoy!

How would you rate this dish?

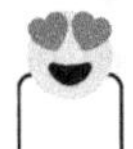 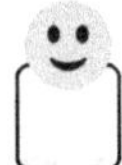  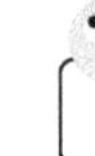 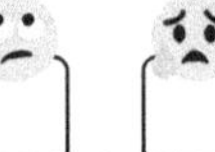

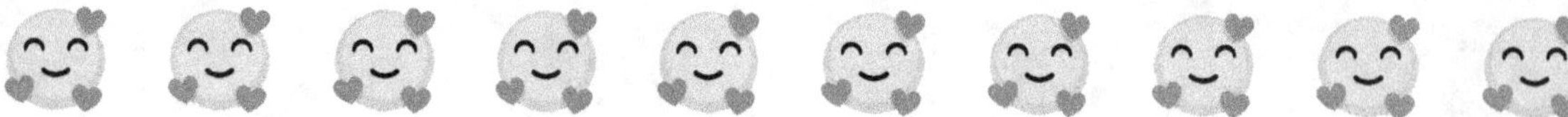

66. Grilled portobello mushrooms with garlic and herbs

 Prep Time :   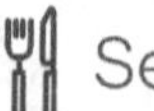 Cook Time :   Servings :

Is this dish easy or difficult for you to make?

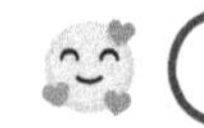 ◯   ◯

Write 5 ....
friends
with   ....
whom
you   ....
want to
share   ....
this
dish   ....

INGREDIENTS

- 4 large portobello mushroom caps, stems removed
- 2 tbsp olive oil
- 3 cloves garlic, minced
- 2 tbsp chopped fresh parsley
- 1 tbsp chopped fresh thyme
- 1 tbsp chopped fresh rosemary
- Salt and pepper to taste

1. Preheat grill or grill pan to medium-high heat.

2. In a small bowl, combine the olive oil, minced garlic, parsley, thyme, and rosemary. Season with salt and pepper.

3. Brush the portobello mushroom caps all over with the garlic-herb oil mixture.

4. Grill the mushrooms for 4-5 minutes per side, until tender and lightly charred.

5. Transfer the grilled portobello mushrooms to a serving plate.

6. Drizzle any remaining garlic-herb oil over the top of the mushrooms. Serve warm.

These grilled portobello mushrooms are a great fertility-supporting dish:

- Portobello mushrooms are a good source of selenium, an important mineral for male fertility.
- Garlic contains allicin, a compound that may help improve sperm quality.
- Herbs like parsley, thyme, and rosemary are rich in antioxidants and have anti-inflammatory properties.
- Olive oil provides healthy monounsaturated fats that can support hormone balance.

The combination of nutrient-dense mushrooms, aromatic herbs, and anti-inflammatory fats makes this a wonderful option for couples trying to conceive. The grilled preparation also adds a delicious, smoky flavor.

Feel free to adjust the herb blend to your taste preferences. These mushrooms can be served as a main dish or a side. Enjoy!

How would you rate this dish?

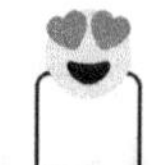 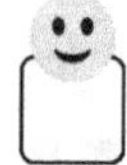 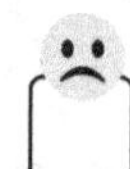 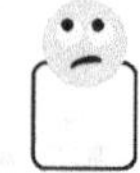 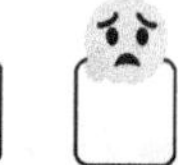

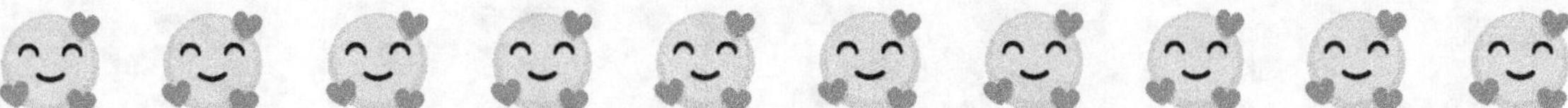

67. Chickpea and vegetable tagine with couscous

 Prep Time :   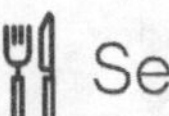 Cook Time :   Servings :

Is this dish easy or difficult for you to make?

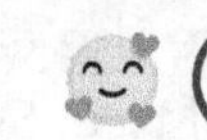 ◯   ◯

Write 5 ....
friends
with   ....
whom
you   ....
want to
share ....
this
dish   ....

INGREDIENTS

For the Tagine:
- 1 tbsp olive oil
- 1 onion, diced
- 3 cloves garlic, minced
- 1 tsp ground cumin
- 1 tsp ground coriander
- 1 tsp paprika
- 1/2 tsp ground cinnamon
- 1/4 tsp cayenne pepper (optional)
- 1 (15 oz) can chickpeas, drained and rinsed
- 1 (14 oz) can diced tomatoes
- 2 cups diced vegetables (such as carrots, zucchini, bell peppers)
- 1 cup vegetable broth
- Salt and pepper to taste
- Chopped cilantro for garnish

For the Couscous:
- 1 cup uncooked couscous
- 1 cup boiling water
- 1 tbsp olive oil
- Salt to taste

How would you rate this dish?

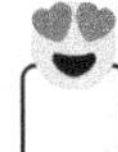 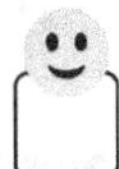 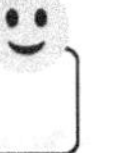 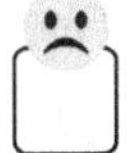 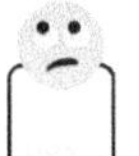 

1. In a large skillet or tagine pot, heat the olive oil over medium heat. Add the onion and sauté for 3-4 minutes until translucent.

2. Stir in the garlic, cumin, coriander, paprika, cinnamon, and cayenne (if using). Cook for 1 minute until fragrant.

3. Add the chickpeas, diced tomatoes, mixed vegetables, and vegetable broth. Bring to a simmer, then reduce heat and let the tagine simmer for 20-25 minutes, until the vegetables are tender.

4. Season the tagine with salt and pepper to taste.

5. While the tagine is simmering, prepare the couscous. In a medium bowl, combine the couscous, boiling water, olive oil, and a pinch of salt. Cover and let sit for 5 minutes, then fluff with a fork.

6. Serve the chickpea and vegetable tagine over the prepared couscous. Garnish with chopped cilantro.

This Moroccan-inspired tagine is packed with fertility-supporting nutrients:

- Chickpeas are a good source of protein, fiber, and folate.
- Vegetables like carrots, zucchini, and bell peppers provide antioxidants, vitamins, and minerals.
- Spices like cumin, coriander, and cinnamon have anti-inflammatory properties.
- Couscous is a whole grain that's high in B vitamins.

The combination of protein, complex carbs, and nutrient-dense vegetables makes this a nourishing and delicious meal for couples trying to conceive. Adjust the spices to your taste preferences. Enjoy!

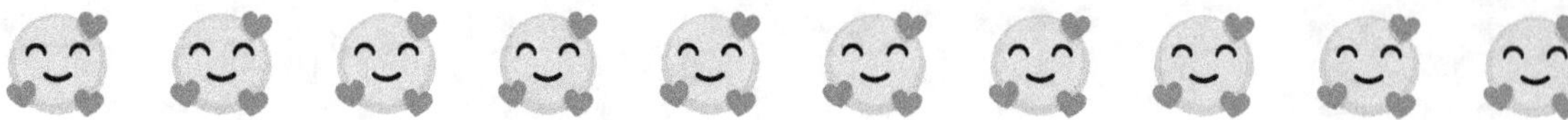

68. Cauliflower rice with peas and carrots

Prep Time :　　Cook Time :　　Servings :

Is this dish easy or difficult for you to make?

 ◯　　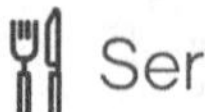 ◯

Write 5 ....
friends
with ....
whom
you ....
want to
share ....
this
dish ....

INGREDIENTS

- 1 head of cauliflower, cut into florets
- 1 tbsp olive oil
- 1 cup frozen peas
- 1 cup diced carrots
- 2 cloves garlic, minced
- 1 tsp ground cumin
- 1 tsp ground coriander
- Salt and pepper to taste
- Chopped fresh parsley for garnish (optional)

1. In a food processor, pulse the cauliflower florets until they resemble the texture of rice. Set aside.

2. In a large skillet, heat the olive oil over medium heat. Add the diced carrots and sauté for 3-4 minutes until starting to soften.

3. Add the frozen peas, minced garlic, cumin, and coriander. Cook for 1-2 minutes until fragrant.

4. Add the riced cauliflower to the skillet and stir to combine. Cook for 5-7 minutes, stirring occasionally, until the cauliflower is tender.

5. Season the cauliflower rice with salt and pepper to taste.

6. Serve the cauliflower rice warm, garnished with chopped fresh parsley if desired.

This cauliflower rice dish is a great fertility-supporting meal:

- Cauliflower is a cruciferous vegetable that's rich in antioxidants, folate, and fiber.
- Peas are a good source of zinc, which is important for male fertility.
- Carrots contain beta-carotene, an antioxidant that may help protect sperm.
- Garlic, cumin, and coriander have anti-inflammatory properties that can improve blood flow.
- Parsley is a natural diuretic and can help flush out toxins.

The combination of nutrient-dense vegetables, aromatic spices, and healthy fats from the olive oil makes this cauliflower rice a great choice for couples trying to conceive. It can be served as a main dish or a side.

How would you rate this dish?

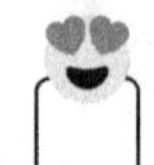 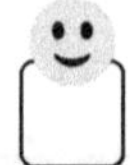 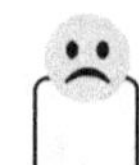 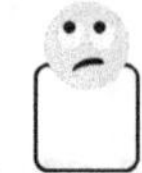 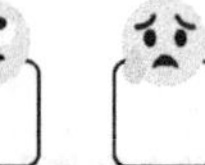

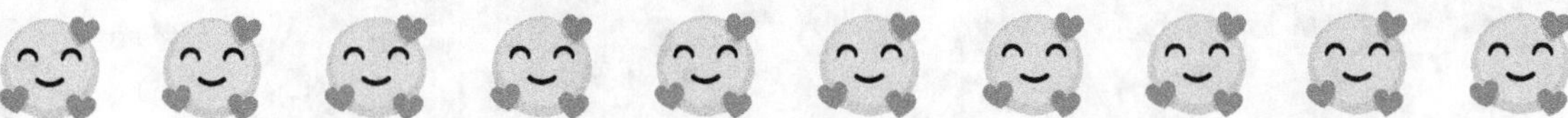

69. Sweet potato and black bean enchiladas

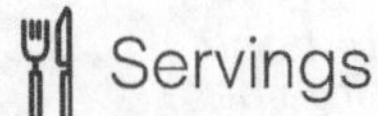

Is this dish easy or difficult for you to make?

Write 5 friends with whom you want to share this dish ....

INGREDIENTS

- 2 medium sweet potatoes, peeled and diced
- 1 (15 oz) can black beans, drained and rinsed
- 1 cup frozen corn kernels
- 1 tsp ground cumin
- 1 tsp chili powder
- Salt and pepper to taste
- 8-10 corn tortillas
- 1 (15 oz) can red enchilada sauce
- 1 cup shredded Monterey Jack or cheddar cheese

1. Preheat oven to 375°F. Grease a 9x13 inch baking dish.

2. In a large skillet, sauté the diced sweet potatoes over medium heat until tender, about 8-10 minutes.

3. Add the black beans, frozen corn, cumin, chili powder, and a pinch of salt and pepper. Stir to combine and cook for 2-3 minutes more.

4. Spread 1/4 cup of the enchilada sauce in the bottom of the prepared baking dish.

5. Warm the corn tortillas according to package instructions. Spoon about 1/4 cup of the sweet potato and black bean mixture onto each tortilla. Roll up the tortillas and place seam-side down in the baking dish.

6. Pour the remaining enchilada sauce over the top of the enchiladas. Sprinkle the shredded cheese evenly over the top.

7. Bake for 20-25 minutes, until the cheese is melted and bubbly. Serve warm, garnished with chopped cilantro if desired.

This sweet potato and black bean enchilada dish is packed with fertility-supporting nutrients:

- Sweet potatoes are rich in beta-carotene, an antioxidant that may help protect sperm.
- Black beans provide protein, fiber, and folate, all important for fertility.
- Corn contains antioxidants like lutein and zeaxanthin that can improve sperm quality.
- Cheese is a good source of zinc, which is crucial for male fertility.
- Cumin and chili powder have anti-inflammatory properties.

How would you rate this dish?

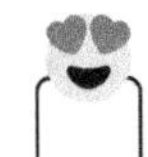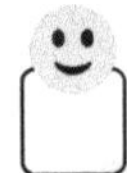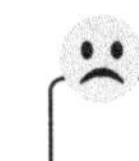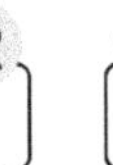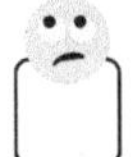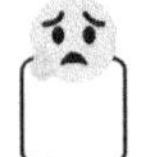

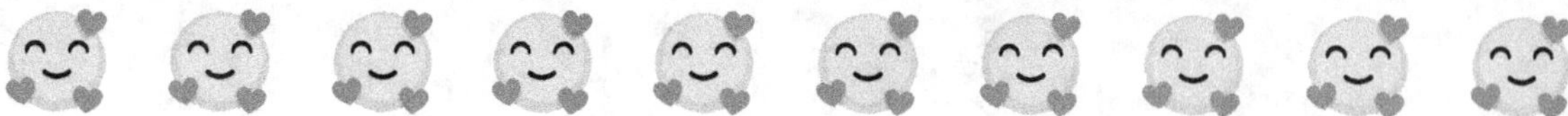

70. Spinach and ricotta stuffed shells

Let's do that and fill in the time here

Prep Time : Cook Time : Servings :

Is this dish easy or difficult for you to make?

 ◯    ◯

Write 5 friends with whom you want to share this dish ....

INGREDIENTS

- 12 jumbo pasta shells
- 1 (15 oz) container ricotta cheese
- 1 cup shredded mozzarella cheese, divided
- 1/2 cup grated Parmesan cheese
- 1 (10 oz) package frozen chopped spinach, thawed and squeezed dry
- 1 egg
- 2 cloves garlic, minced
- 1 tsp dried oregano
- 1/4 tsp nutmeg
- Salt and pepper to taste
- 1 (24 oz) jar marinara sauce

1. Preheat oven to 375°F. Grease a 9x13 inch baking dish.

2. Cook the pasta shells according to package instructions until al dente. Drain and set aside.

3. In a large bowl, mix together the ricotta, 1/2 cup of the mozzarella, Parmesan, spinach, egg, garlic, oregano, nutmeg, salt, and pepper.

4. Stuff each cooked pasta shell with a heaping spoonful of the ricotta-spinach mixture.

5. Spread 1/2 cup of the marinara sauce in the bottom of the prepared baking dish. Arrange the stuffed shells in a single layer.

6. Pour the remaining marinara sauce over the top of the shells. Sprinkle the remaining 1/2 cup of mozzarella cheese over the top.

7. Bake for 25-30 minutes, until the cheese is melted and bubbly. Let cool for 5 minutes before serving.

This spinach and ricotta stuffed shells dish is a great fertility-supporting meal:

- Spinach is rich in folate, an important nutrient for both male and female fertility.
- Ricotta cheese provides protein and zinc, which are crucial for sperm health.
- Mozzarella and Parmesan cheeses also contain zinc and other fertility-boosting minerals.
- Garlic and oregano have anti-inflammatory properties that can improve blood flow.
- The tomato-based marinara sauce contains lycopene, an antioxidant that may help protect sperm.

How would you rate this dish?

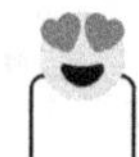 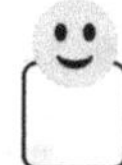 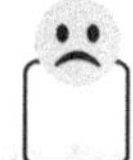 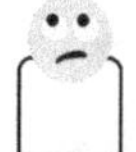 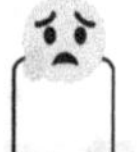

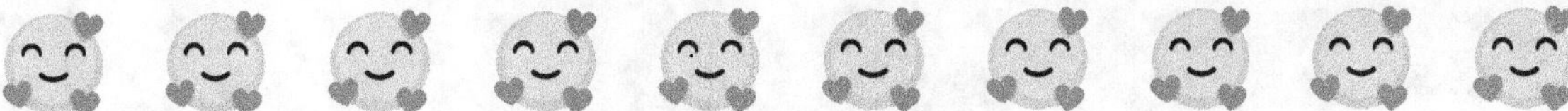

71. Baked tilapia with lemon and capers

Let's do that and fill in the time here

Prep Time :   Cook Time :   Servings :

Is this dish easy or difficult for you to make?

 ○   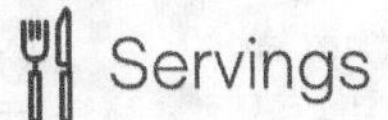 ○

Write 5 ....
friends
with ....
whom
you ....
want to
share ....
this
dish ....

INGREDIENTS

- 4 tilapia fillets (about 1 lb total)
- 2 tbsp olive oil
- 2 tbsp lemon juice
- 2 tbsp capers, drained
- 2 cloves garlic, minced
- 1 tsp dried parsley
- Salt and pepper to taste
- Lemon wedges for serving

How would you rate this dish?

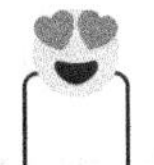 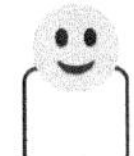 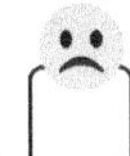 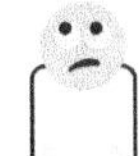 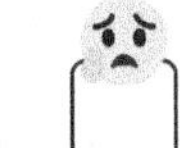

1. Preheat oven to 400°F. Grease a baking dish with nonstick cooking spray.

2. Place the tilapia fillets in the prepared baking dish.

3. In a small bowl, whisk together the olive oil, lemon juice, capers, garlic, and dried parsley. Season with salt and pepper.

4. Pour the lemon-caper sauce over the tilapia fillets, making sure to evenly coat the fish.

5. Bake for 15-18 minutes, until the tilapia is opaque and flakes easily with a fork.

6. Serve the baked tilapia warm, with lemon wedges on the side.

This baked tilapia dish is a great fertility-supporting meal:

- Tilapia is a lean source of protein and contains omega-3 fatty acids, which are important for sperm health.
- Lemon juice is high in vitamin C, an antioxidant that can help improve sperm quality.
- Capers are a good source of zinc, a mineral crucial for male fertility.
- Garlic has anti-inflammatory properties that can improve blood flow.
- Parsley is a natural diuretic and can help flush out toxIns.

The combination of protein-rich fish, citrus, and fertility-boosting herbs and spices makes this a wonderful option for couples trying to conceive. Serve it with a side of roasted vegetables or a fresh salad for a complete, nourishing meal.

Enjoy this delicious and fertility-supporting baked tilapia!

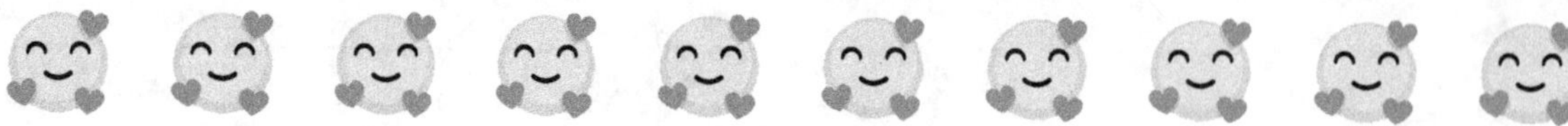

72. Grilled swordfish with a mango salsa

Prep Time :   Cook Time :   Servings :

Is this dish easy or difficult for you to make?

 ◯   ◯

Write 5 ....
friends
with ....
whom
you ....
want to
share ....
this
dish ....

INGREDIENTS

For the Mango Salsa:
- 1 ripe mango, diced
- 1/2 red onion, finely chopped
- 1 jalapeño, seeded and finely chopped
- 1/4 cup chopped fresh cilantro
- 2 tbsp lime juice
- 1 tsp olive oil
- Salt and pepper to taste

For the Swordfish:
- 4 (6 oz) swordfish steaks
- 2 tbsp olive oil
- 1 tsp chili powder
- 1 tsp ground cumin
- Salt and pepper to taste

1. Make the mango salsa: In a medium bowl, combine the diced mango, red onion, jalapeño, cilantro, lime juice, and olive oil. Season with salt and pepper. Cover and refrigerate until ready to serve.

2. Preheat grill or grill pan to medium-high heat.

3. Pat the swordfish steaks dry and brush both sides with olive oil. Season with chili powder, cumin, salt, and pepper.

4. Grill the swordfish for 4-5 minutes per side, until opaque and cooked through.

5. Transfer the grilled swordfish to plates and top with the chilled mango salsa. Serve immediately.

This grilled swordfish dish is packed with fertility-supporting nutrients:

- Swordfish is a great source of omega-3 fatty acids, which are important for sperm health.
- Mangoes are rich in vitamin C, an antioxidant that can help improve sperm quality.
- Jalapeños contain capsaicin, a compound that may help increase blood flow.
- Cilantro is a natural diuretic and can help flush out toxins.
- Olive oil provides healthy monounsaturated fats that support hormone balance.

The combination of nutrient-dense fish, tropical fruit, and anti-inflammatory spices makes this a wonderful meal for couples trying to conceive. The fresh, vibrant mango salsa complements the grilled swordfish perfectly.

Enjoy this fertility-boosting dish!

How would you rate this dish?

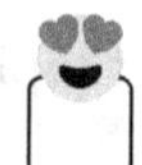 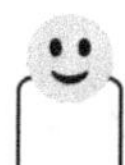 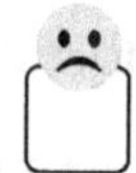 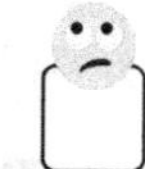 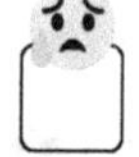

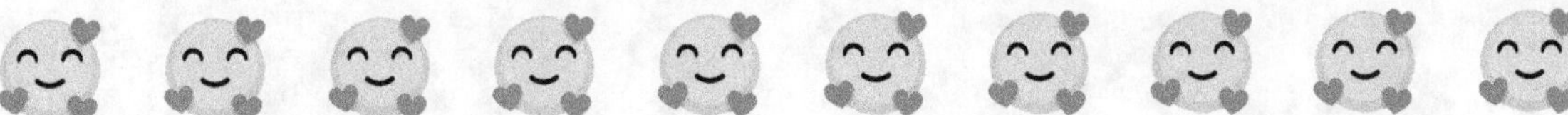

73. Shrimp and avocado salad with mixed greens

Prep Time :   Cook Time :   Servings :

Is this dish easy or difficult for you to make?

 ◯   😊 ◯

Write 5 friends with whom you want to share this dish ....

INGREDIENTS

- 1 lb cooked shrimp, peeled and deveined
- 1 avocado, diced
- 1 cup cherry tomatoes, halved
- 1/2 red onion, thinly sliced
- 5 oz mixed greens (such as spinach, arugula, and kale)
- 2 tbsp olive oil
- 2 tbsp balsamic vinegar
- 1 tsp Dijon mustard
- 1 tsp honey
- Salt and pepper to taste

How would you rate this dish?

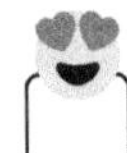  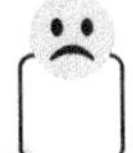 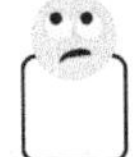 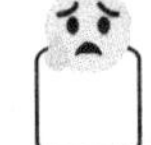

1. In a large salad bowl, combine the cooked shrimp, diced avocado, cherry tomatoes, and red onion slices.

2. In a small bowl, whisk together the olive oil, balsamic vinegar, Dijon mustard, and honey. Season with salt and pepper.

3. Add the mixed greens to the salad bowl and drizzle the dressing over the top. Toss gently to coat.

4. Serve the shrimp and avocado salad Immediately.

This salad is packed with fertility-supporting nutrients:

- Shrimp is a good source of protein, zinc, and selenium, all important for male fertility.

- Avocado is rich in healthy monounsaturated fats that can help support hormone balance.

- Mixed greens like spinach and arugula are high in folate, a crucial nutrient for both male and female fertility.

- Cherry tomatoes contain lycopene, an antioxidant that may help protect sperm.

- Olive oil and balsamic vinegar provide anti-inflammatory benefits.

The combination of protein-rich shrimp, nutrient-dense greens, healthy fats, and antioxidants makes this a wonderful salad for couples trying to conceive. It can be enjoyed as a main dish or a side.

Feel free to adjust the amounts of any ingredients to suit your taste preferences. Enjoy this fertility-boosting salad!

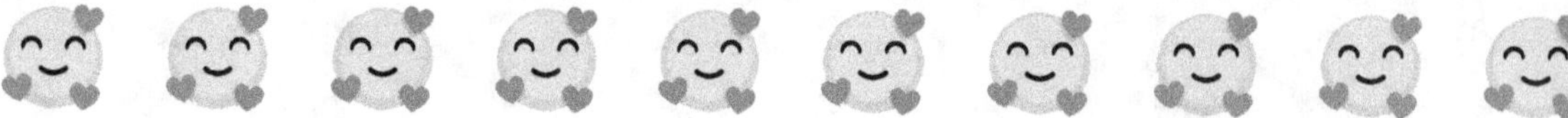

74. Baked haddock with a breadcrumb crust

Prep Time :   Cook Time :   Servings :

Is this dish easy or difficult for you to make?

 ◯   ◯

Write 5 friends with whom you want to share this dish

....
....
....
....

INGREDIENTS

- 4 (6 oz) haddock fillets
- 1/2 cup panko breadcrumbs
- 2 tbsp grated Parmesan cheese
- 2 tbsp chopped fresh parsley
- 2 tbsp olive oil, plus more for drizzling
- 1 tbsp lemon juice
- 1 tsp Dijon mustard
- Salt and pepper to taste

How would you rate this dish?

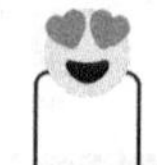 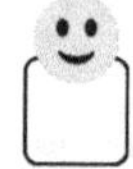  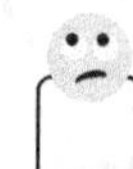 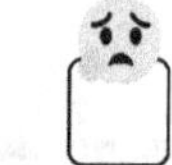

1. Preheat oven to 400°F. Grease a baking dish with nonstick cooking spray.

2. In a shallow bowl, combine the panko breadcrumbs, Parmesan cheese, and chopped parsley.

3. In a small bowl, whisk together the 2 tbsp olive oil, lemon juice, and Dijon mustard. Season with salt and pepper.

4. Place the haddock fillets in the prepared baking dish. Drizzle the oil-lemon mixture over the top of the fish.

5. Sprinkle the breadcrumb mixture evenly over the haddock, pressing gently to adhere.

6. Bake for 15-18 minutes, until the fish is opaque and the breadcrumb topping is golden brown.

7. Serve the baked haddock immediately, garnished with additional chopped parsley if desired.

This baked haddock dish is a great fertility-supporting meal:

- Haddock is a lean, protein-rich fish that's high in omega-3 fatty acids, which are important for sperm health.
- Panko breadcrumbs provide a crunchy texture and complex carbohydrates.
- Parmesan cheese is a good source of zinc, a crucial mineral for male fertility.
- Parsley is a natural diuretic and can help flush out toxins.
- Lemon juice and Dijon mustard add flavor and provide antioxidant benefits.
- Olive oil contains healthy monounsaturated fats that support hormone balance.

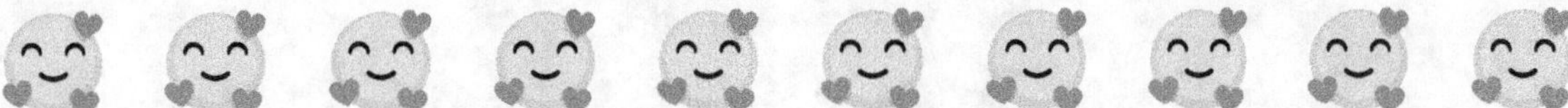

75. Sardine and arugula salad with lemon dressing

 Prep Time :   Cook Time :   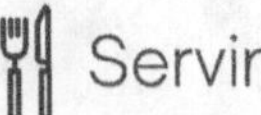 Servings :

Is this dish easy or difficult for you to make?

Write 5 friends with whom you want to share this dish ....

INGREDIENTS

- 5 oz baby arugula
- 1 (4 oz) can sardines in olive oil, drained and flaked
- 1 avocado, diced
- 1/4 cup sliced almonds
- 2 tbsp olive oil
- 2 tbsp lemon juice
- 1 tsp Dijon mustard
- 1 tsp honey
- Salt and pepper to taste

How would you rate this dish?

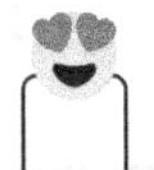 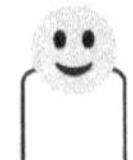 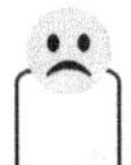 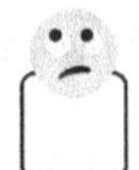 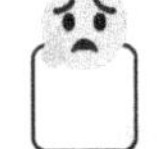

1. In a large salad bowl, combine the baby arugula, flaked sardines, diced avocado, and sliced almonds.

2. In a small bowl, whisk together the olive oil, lemon juice, Dijon mustard, and honey. Season with salt and pepper.

3. Drizzle the lemon dressing over the salad and toss gently to coat. Serve the sardine and arugula salad immediately.

This salad is packed with fertility-supporting nutrients:

- Sardines are an excellent source of omega-3 fatty acids, which are important for sperm health.

- Arugula is rich in folate, a crucial nutrient for both male and female fertility.

- Avocado provides healthy monounsaturated fats that can help support hormone balance.

- Almonds contain zinc, vitamin E, and other antioxidants that may improve sperm quality.

- Lemon juice is high in vitamin C, which can help protect sperm.

- Olive oil and Dijon mustard have anti-inflammatory properties.

The combination of nutrient-dense greens, protein-rich sardines, healthy fats, and antioxidants makes this a wonderful salad for couples trying to conceive. It can be enjoyed as a main dish or a side.

Feel free to adjust the amounts of any ingredients to suit your taste preferences. Enjoy this fertility-boosting salad!

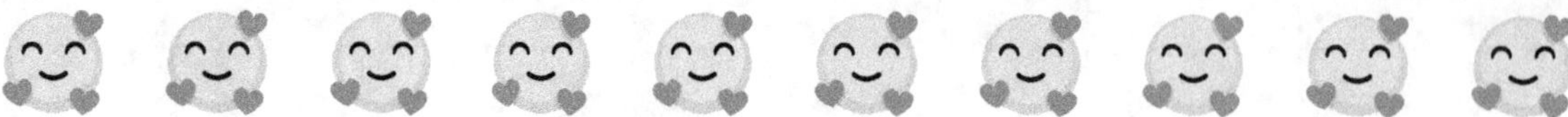

76. Mackerel with a tomato and onion relish

 Prep Time :   Cook Time :   Servings :

Is this dish easy or difficult for you to make?

Write 5 ....
friends
with   ....
whom
you   ....
want to
share   ....
this
dish   ....

INGREDIENTS

For the Relish:
- 2 tomatoes, diced
- 1/2 red onion, finely chopped
- 2 tbsp chopped fresh parsley
- 1 tbsp olive oil
- 1 tbsp red wine vinegar
- 1 tsp honey
- Salt and pepper to taste

For the Mackerel:
- 4 (6 oz) mackerel fillets
- 1 tbsp olive oil
- 1 tsp paprika
- Salt and pepper to taste

How would you rate this dish?

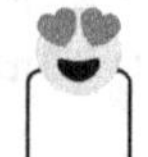 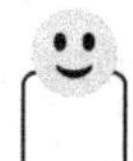  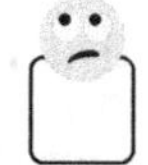 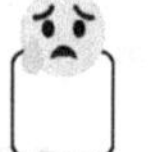

1. Make the tomato and onion relish: In a medium bowl, combine the diced tomatoes, chopped red onion, parsley, olive oil, red wine vinegar, and honey. Season with salt and pepper. Cover and refrigerate until ready to serve.

2. Preheat oven to 400°F. Line a baking sheet with parchment paper.

3. Pat the mackerel fillets dry and place them on the prepared baking sheet. Drizzle with the 1 tbsp olive oil and sprinkle with paprika, salt, and pepper.

4. Roast the mackerel for 12-15 minutes, until cooked through and flaky.

5. Transfer the roasted mackerel fillets to plates and top with the chilled tomato and onion relish. Serve immediately.

This mackerel dish is packed with fertility-supporting nutrients:

- Mackerel is an oily fish that's rich in omega-3 fatty acids, which are important for sperm health.
- Tomatoes contain lycopene, an antioxidant that may help protect sperm.
- Red onion is a good source of quercetin, a flavonoid with anti-inflammatory properties.
- Parsley is a natural diuretic and can help flush out toxins.
- Olive oil and vinegar provide healthy fats and antioxidants.
- Paprika contains capsaicin, a compound that may help increase blood flow.

The combination of nutrient-dense fish, fresh vegetables, and anti-inflammatory ingredients makes this a wonderful meal for couples trying to conceive.

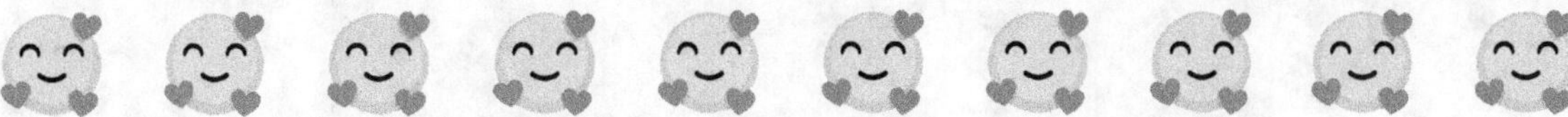

77. Tuna steak with a wasabi glaze

 Prep Time :   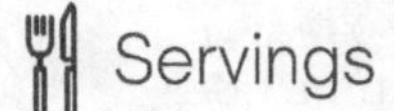 Cook Time :   Servings :

Is this dish easy or difficult for you to make?

Write 5 ....
friends
with ....
whom
you ....
want to
share ....
this
dish ....

INGREDIENTS

- 4 (6 oz) tuna steaks
- 2 tbsp soy sauce
- 2 tbsp rice vinegar
- 1 tbsp honey
- 1-2 tsp prepared wasabi paste
- 1 tbsp sesame oil
- 1 tbsp vegetable oil
- Salt and pepper to taste
- Sesame seeds for garnish (optional)

How would you rate this dish?

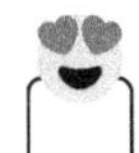   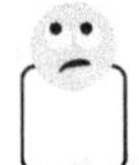 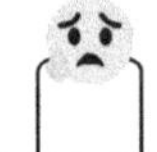

1. In a small bowl, whisk together the soy sauce, rice vinegar, honey, and 1-2 tsp of wasabi paste (depending on your desired level of heat). Set aside.

2. Heat the sesame oil and vegetable oil in a large skillet or grill pan over medium-high heat.

3. Season the tuna steaks with salt and pepper on both sides.

4. Sear the tuna steaks for 2-3 minutes per side, until the outside is lightly browned but the center is still pink and rare.

5. Transfer the tuna steaks to a plate and brush the tops generously with the wasabi glaze.

6. Serve the tuna steaks immediately, garnished with sesame seeds if desired.

This tuna dish is packed with fertility-supporting nutrients:

- Tuna is an excellent source of omega-3 fatty acids, which are important for sperm health.
- Wasabi contains allyl isothiocyanate, a compound that may help increase blood flow.
- Soy sauce and rice vinegar provide antioxidants and anti-inflammatory benefits.
- Honey is a natural source of carbohydrates and contains trace minerals.
- Sesame oil and seeds are rich in zinc, a crucial mineral for male fertility.

The combination of nutrient-dense fish, spicy wasabi, and healthy fats makes this a wonderful meal for couples trying to conceive. The quick searing method helps preserve the tuna's delicate texture and flavor.

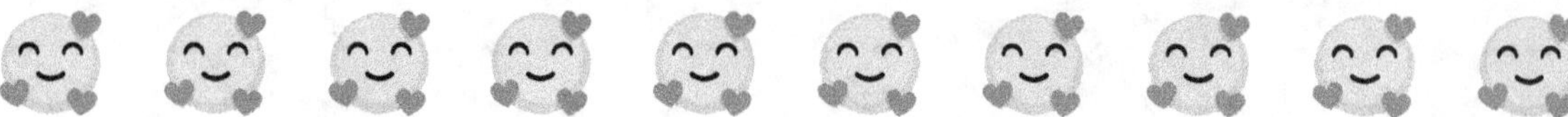

78. Salmon cakes with a dill yogurt sauce

 Prep Time :   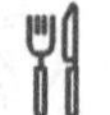 Cook Time :   Servings :

Is this dish easy or difficult for you to make?

⭕   ⭕

Write 5 friends with whom you want to share this dish

....

....

....

....

....

INGREDIENTS

For the Salmon Cakes:
- 1 (15 oz) can wild-caught salmon, drained and flaked
- 1 egg, lightly beaten
- 1/2 cup panko breadcrumbs
- 2 tbsp chopped fresh dill
- 1 tbsp Dijon mustard
- 1 tbsp lemon juice
- Salt and pepper to taste
- 2 tbsp olive oil for cooking

For the Dill Yogurt Sauce:
- 1 cup plain Greek yogurt
- 2 tbsp chopped fresh dill
- 1 tbsp lemon juice
- 1 tsp honey
- Salt and pepper to taste

How would you rate this dish?

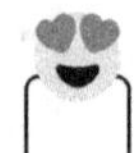 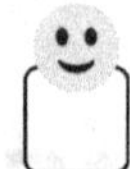 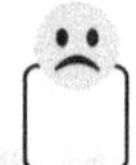 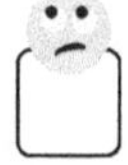 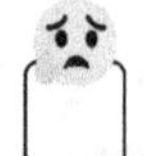

1. In a medium bowl, gently mix together the flaked salmon, egg, panko breadcrumbs, 2 tbsp dill, Dijon mustard, and lemon juice. Season with salt and pepper.

2. Form the salmon mixture into 8 small patties, about 1/2 inch thick.

3. In a large skillet, heat the 2 tbsp olive oil over medium heat. Cook the salmon cakes for 3-4 minutes per side, until golden brown.

4. Meanwhile, make the dill yogurt sauce. In a small bowl, stir together the Greek yogurt, 2 tbsp dill, lemon juice, honey, salt, and pepper.

5. Serve the salmon cakes warm, topped with the dill yogurt sauce.

This salmon cake dish is packed with fertility-supporting nutrients:

- Salmon is an excellent source of omega-3 fatty acids, which are important for sperm health.
- Eggs provide high-quality protein and vitamins like B12 and D.
- Panko breadcrumbs are a whole grain that provides complex carbs.
- Dill is a natural diuretic and can help flush out toxins.
- Greek yogurt is rich in protein and probiotics, which may improve gut health.
- Lemon juice and honey provide antioxidants and anti-inflammatory benefits.

The combination of nutrient-dense salmon, whole grains, and probiotic-rich yogurt makes this a wonderful meal for couples trying to conceive. The dill yogurt sauce adds a refreshing, herbal element.

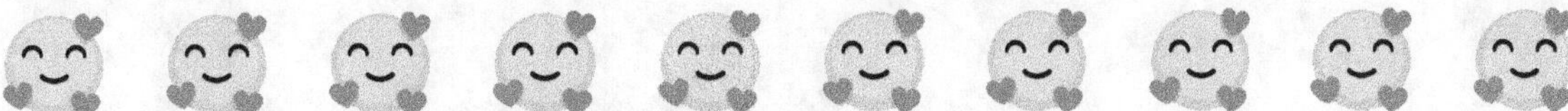

79. Crab-stuffed mushrooms

Let's do that and fill in the time here ✅ Prep Time :   🕐 Cook Time :   🍴 Servings :

Is this dish easy or difficult for you to make?

 ◯   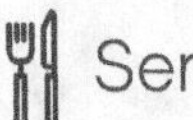 ◯

Write 5 friends with whom you want to share this dish

....

....

....

....

....

INGREDIENTS

- 12 large mushrooms, stems removed and finely chopped
- 1 tbsp olive oil
- 1/2 cup lump crabmeat, picked over for shells
- 2 tbsp grated Parmesan cheese
- 2 tbsp panko breadcrumbs
- 2 tbsp chopped fresh parsley
- 1 tbsp lemon juice
- 1 tsp Dijon mustard
- Salt and pepper to taste

1. Preheat oven to 375°F. Grease a baking sheet or oven-safe dish.

2. In a skillet, heat the olive oil over medium heat. Add the finely chopped mushroom stems and sauté for 3-4 minutes until softened.

3. Remove the skillet from heat and let the mushroom stems cool slightly. Then, in a medium bowl, mix the sautéed mushroom stems with the crabmeat, Parmesan, panko, parsley, lemon juice, and Dijon mustard. Season with salt and pepper.

4. Stuff the mushroom caps evenly with the crab mixture, packing it in gently.

5. Arrange the stuffed mushrooms on the prepared baking sheet or dish.

6. Bake for 12-15 minutes, until the mushrooms are tender and the filling is hot. Serve the crab-stuffed mushrooms warm.

These crab-stuffed mushrooms are a great fertility-supporting appetizer or side dish:

- Crabmeat is a good source of zinc, a crucial mineral for male fertility.
- Mushrooms contain selenium, an antioxidant that may help protect sperm.
- Parmesan cheese provides protein and additional zinc.
- Panko breadcrumbs are a whole grain that offers complex carbs.
- Parsley is a natural diuretic and can help flush out toxins.
- Lemon juice and Dijon mustard add anti-inflammatory benefits.

How would you rate this dish?

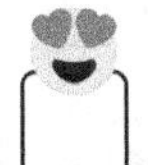 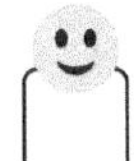 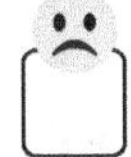 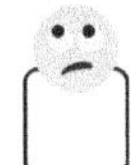 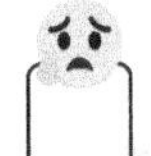

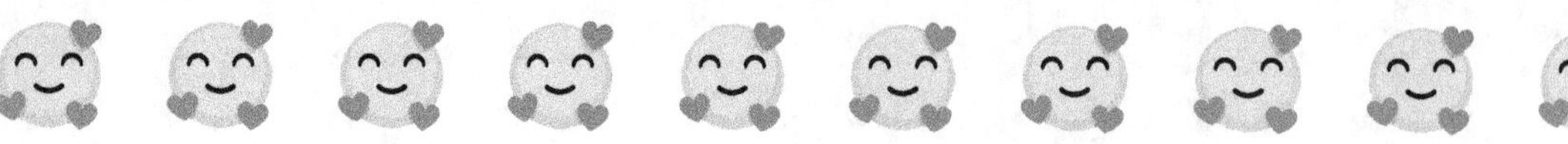

80. Seafood paella with brown rice

 *Let's do that and fill in the time here* 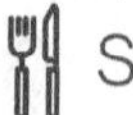 Prep Time :   Cook Time :   Servings :

Is this dish easy or difficult for you to make?

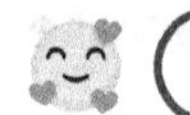 ◯   ◯

Write 5 ....
friends
with   ....
whom
you   ....
want to
share   ....
this
dish   ....

INGREDIENTS

- 1 cup short-grain brown rice
- 2 cups low-sodium chicken or vegetable broth
- 1 tbsp olive oil
- 1 onion, diced
- 3 cloves garlic, minced
- 1 tsp smoked paprika
- 1/2 tsp saffron threads
- 1 cup diced tomatoes
- 1 lb shrimp, peeled and deveined
- 1 lb mussels, scrubbed and debearded
- 1 lb calamari, bodies sliced into rings
- 1 cup frozen peas
- 2 tbsp chopped fresh parsley
- Salt and pepper to taste

1. In a medium saucepan, bring the brown rice and broth to a boil. Reduce heat, cover and simmer for 40-45 minutes until rice is tender. Fluff with a fork.

2. In a large skillet or paella pan, heat the olive oil over medium heat. Add the onion and cook for 5 minutes until translucent. Add the garlic, paprika and saffron and cook for 1 minute.

3. Stir in the tomatoes and cook for 2-3 minutes.

4. Add the shrimp, mussels and calamari. Cover and cook for 5-7 minutes until the seafood is cooked through.

5. Stir in the cooked brown rice and peas. Season with salt and pepper.

6. Garnish with fresh parsley before serving.

Enjoy your healthy and flavorful seafood paella!

How would you rate this dish?

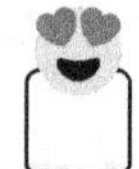 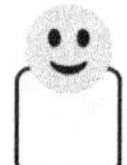 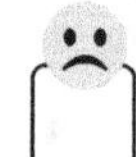 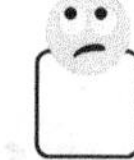 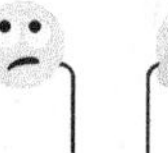 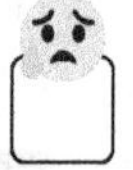

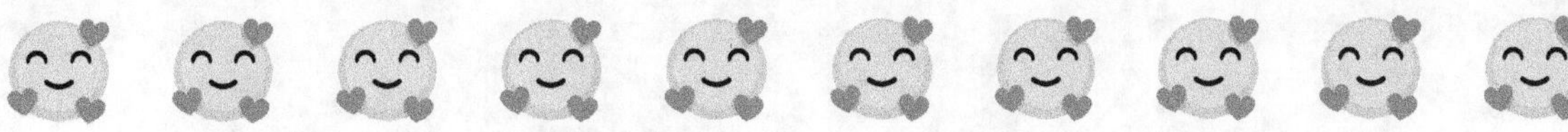

81. Roast chicken with rosemary and garlic

Let's do that and fill in the time here

 Prep Time :   Cook Time :   Servings :

Is this dish easy or difficult for you to make?

○   ○

Write 5 friends with whom you want to share this dish

INGREDIENTS

- 1 whole chicken (4-5 lbs)
- 6 cloves garlic, minced
- 2 tbsp fresh rosemary, chopped
- 2 tbsp olive oil
- 1 tsp sea salt
- 1/2 tsp black pepper

For the Fertility-Boosting Sides:
- 1 lb roasted sweet potatoes
- 1 cup sautéed spinach with garlic
- 1/2 cup quinoa

1. Preheat oven to 400°F. Pat the chicken dry with paper towels.

2. In a small bowl, mix together the minced garlic, chopped rosemary, olive oil, salt and pepper.

3. Rub the garlic-rosemary mixture all over the outside of the chicken, making sure to get it under the skin as well.

4. Place the chicken in a roasting pan and roast for 1 to 1 1/2 hours, until the juices run clear when the thigh is pierced. The internal temperature should reach 165°F.

5. Let the chicken rest for 10 minutes before carving.

For the Fertility-Boosting Sides:

1. Roast the sweet potatoes at 400°F for 30-40 minutes until tender.

2. Sauté the spinach with 2 cloves minced garlic in a skillet with a bit of olive oil until wilted.

3. Cook the quinoa according to package instructions.

Serve the roast chicken with the sweet potatoes, sautéed spinach, and quinoa. The combination of nutrients in this meal can help support fertility in both men and women.

Enjoy!

How would you rate this dish?

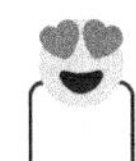 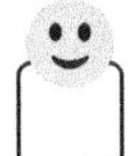 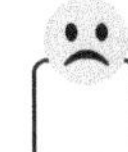 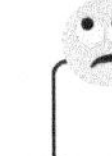 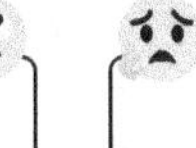

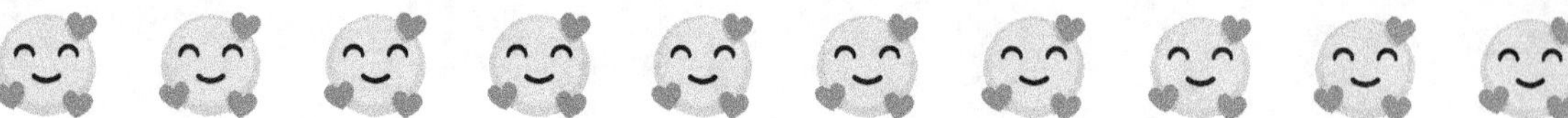

82. Chicken stir-fry with broccoli and cashews

Prep Time :   Cook Time :   Servings :

Is this dish easy or difficult for you to make?

 ○    ○

Write 5 friends with whom you want to share this dish

....

....

....

....

....

INGREDIENTS

- 1 lb boneless, skinless chicken breasts, cut into 1-inch pieces
- 2 tbsp sesame oil
- 3 cloves garlic, minced
- 1 tbsp grated fresh ginger
- 1 head broccoli, cut into florets
- 1 cup raw cashews
- 2 tbsp low-sodium soy sauce
- 1 tbsp rice vinegar
- 1 tsp honey
- 1/4 tsp red pepper flakes (optional)
- Salt and pepper to taste
- Cooked brown rice, for serving

1. Heat the sesame oil in a large skillet or wok over medium-high heat. Add the chicken and cook for 5-7 minutes, stirring occasionally, until browned and cooked through. Remove the chicken from the pan and set aside.

2. Add the garlic and ginger to the pan and cook for 1 minute, until fragrant.

3. Add the broccoli florets and cashews to the pan. Stir-fry for 3-5 minutes, until the broccoli is tender-crisp.

4. In a small bowl, whisk together the soy sauce, rice vinegar, honey, and red pepper flakes (if using).

5. Return the cooked chicken to the pan and pour the sauce over the top. Toss everything together and cook for 2-3 minutes, until the sauce has thickened slightly.

6. Season with salt and pepper to taste.

7. Serve the chicken stir-fry over cooked brown rice.

This dish is packed with fertility-boosting nutrients like:
- Chicken - a great source of protein
- Broccoli - high in folate, vitamin C, and antioxidants
- Cashews - rich in zinc, which is important for male fertility
- Brown rice - a complex carb that provides sustained energy

Enjoy this delicious and nutritious stir-fry!

How would you rate this dish?

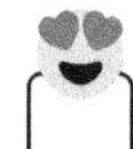 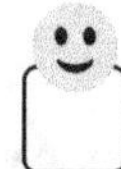 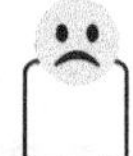 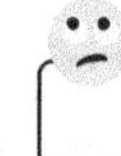 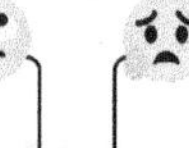

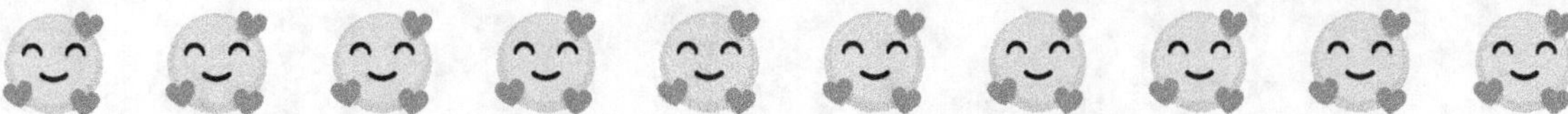

83. Turkey meatballs with marinara sauce

Prep Time :

Cook Time :

Servings :

Is this dish easy or difficult for you to make?

 ◯   ◯

Write 5 friends with whom you want to share this dish

INGREDIENTS

For the Meatballs:
- 1 lb ground turkey
- 1/2 cup whole wheat breadcrumbs
- 1/4 cup grated Parmesan cheese
- 2 cloves garlic, minced
- 1 egg, lightly beaten
- 2 tbsp chopped fresh parsley
- 1 tsp dried oregano
- 1/2 tsp salt
- 1/4 tsp black pepper

For the Marinara Sauce:
- 1 tbsp olive oil
- 1 onion, diced
- 3 cloves garlic, minced
- 1 (28 oz) can crushed tomatoes
- 2 tbsp tomato paste
- 1 tsp dried basil
- 1/2 tsp dried oregano
- 1/4 tsp red pepper flakes (optional)
- Salt and pepper to taste

1. Preheat oven to 400°F. Line a baking sheet with parchment paper.

For the Meatballs:
2. In a large bowl, combine all the meatball ingredients and mix well. Roll the mixture into 1-inch balls and place them on the prepared baking sheet.
3. Bake for 18-20 minutes, until cooked through.

For the Marinara Sauce:
4. In a large saucepan, heat the olive oil over medium heat. Add the onion and cook for 5 minutes until translucent.
5. Add the garlic and cook for 1 minute until fragrant.
6. Stir in the crushed tomatoes, tomato paste, basil, oregano, and red pepper flakes (if using). Season with salt and pepper.
7. Simmer the sauce for 10-15 minutes, until thickened.

To Serve:
8. Add the cooked turkey meatballs to the marinara sauce and gently toss to coat.
9. Serve the meatballs and sauce over whole wheat pasta or zucchini noodles.

This dish is packed with fertility-boosting nutrients like:
- Turkey - a lean protein source
- Whole wheat breadcrumbs - a complex carb
- Parmesan cheese - a good source of calcium
- Tomatoes - rich in the antioxidant lycopene
- Garlic and onions - contain allicin, which may improve sperm quality

Enjoy this delicious and nutritious meal!

How would you rate this dish?

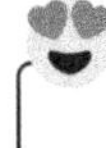 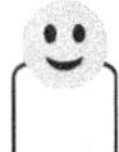 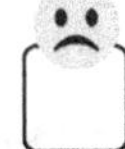 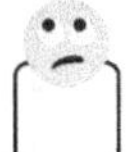 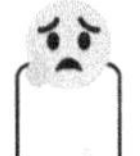

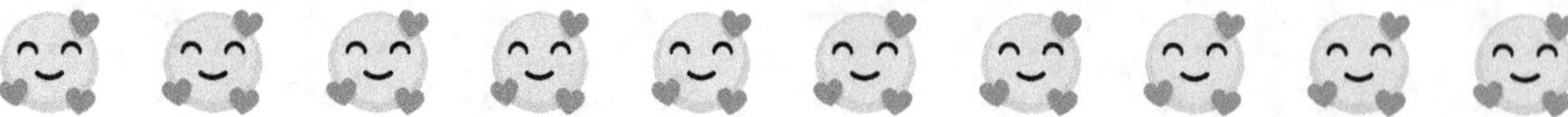

84. Chicken fajitas with bell peppers and onions

Prep Time :   Cook Time :   Servings :

Is this dish easy or difficult for you to make?

 ◯   ◯

Write 5 friends with whom you want to share this dish ....

INGREDIENTS

- 1 lb boneless, skinless chicken breasts, sliced into strips
- 2 bell peppers (any color), sliced
- 1 onion, sliced
- 2 tbsp olive oil
- 2 tsp chili powder
- 1 tsp cumin
- 1 tsp garlic powder
- 1/2 tsp oregano
- 1/4 tsp cayenne pepper (optional)
- Salt and pepper to taste
- 8-10 whole wheat tortillas
- Toppings: avocado, plain Greek yogurt, salsa, cilantro

1. In a large skillet or wok, heat the olive oil over medium-high heat.

2. Add the chicken strips and season with the chili powder, cumin, garlic powder, oregano, cayenne (if using), salt, and pepper. Cook for 5-7 minutes, stirring occasionally, until the chicken is cooked through.

3. Add the sliced bell peppers and onions to the pan. Sauté for 5-7 minutes, until the vegetables are tender-crisp.

4. Warm the whole wheat tortillas according to package instructions.

5. To serve, place some of the chicken and vegetable mixture into each tortilla. Top with desired toppings like avocado, Greek yogurt, salsa, and cilantro.

This dish is packed with fertility-boosting nutrients:

- Chicken - a lean protein source
- Bell peppers - high in vitamin C, which is important for fertility
- Onions - contain allicin, which may improve sperm quality
- Avocado - rich in healthy fats that support hormone production
- Greek yogurt - provides probiotics and calcium

The whole wheat tortillas also provide complex carbs for sustained energy.

Enjoy these delicious and nutritious chicken fajitas!

How would you rate this dish?

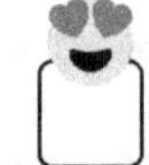 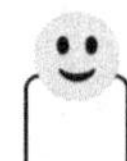  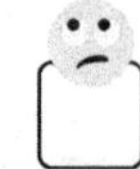 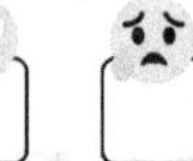 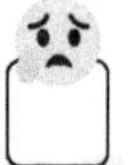

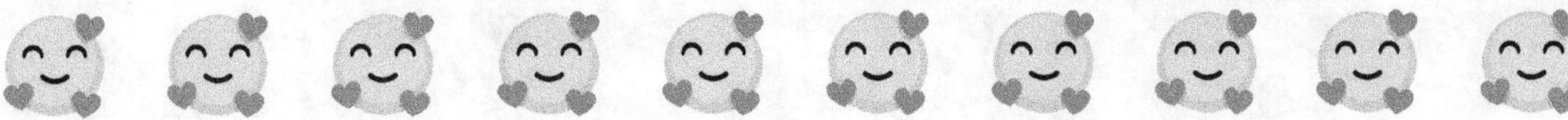

85. Grilled turkey burgers with avocado

Is this dish easy or difficult for you to make?

Write 5 friends with whom you want to share this dish

....

....

....

....

....

INGREDIENTS

- 1 lb ground turkey
- 1/4 cup whole wheat breadcrumbs
- 2 tbsp chopped fresh parsley
- 1 tsp garlic powder
- 1/2 tsp onion powder
- 1/4 tsp cayenne pepper (optional)
- Salt and pepper to taste
- 4 whole wheat burger buns
- 1 avocado, sliced
- Lettuce, tomato, and other desired toppings

For the Fertility-Boosting Sauce:
- 1/2 cup plain Greek yogurt
- 2 tbsp Dijon mustard
- 1 tbsp lemon juice
- 1 tsp honey
- Salt and pepper to taste

1. Preheat grill or grill pan to medium-high heat.

2. In a large bowl, combine the ground turkey, breadcrumbs, parsley, garlic powder, onion powder, cayenne (if using), and a pinch of salt and pepper. Mix well and form into 4 equal-sized patties.

3. Grill the turkey burgers for 5-7 minutes per side, until cooked through.

4. In a small bowl, whisk together the ingredients for the fertility-boosting sauce.

5. Spread the sauce on the bottom buns, then top with the grilled turkey burgers, avocado slices, lettuce, tomato, and any other desired toppings.

6. Place the top buns on the burgers and serve.

This dish is packed with fertility-boosting nutrients:

- Turkey - a lean protein source
- Whole wheat buns - provide complex carbs
- Avocado - rich in healthy fats that support hormone production
- Greek yogurt - provides probiotics and calcium
- Mustard and lemon - contain antioxidants

The combination of these ingredients can help support fertility in both men and women.

Enjoy these delicious and nutritious turkey burgers!

How would you rate this dish?

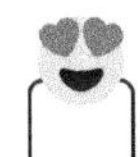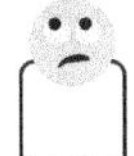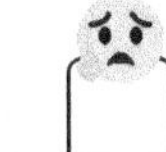

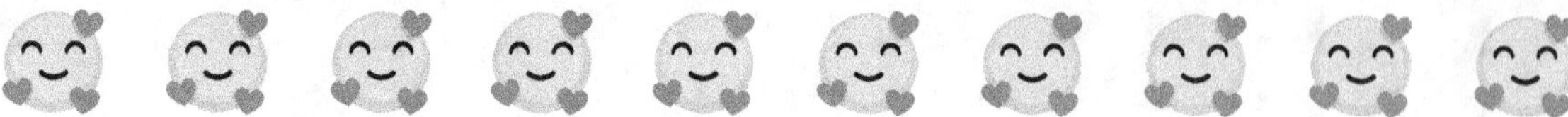

86. Lemon herb chicken breasts with quinoa

Let's do that and fill in the time here  Prep Time :   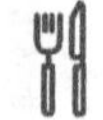 Cook Time :   Servings :

Is this dish easy or difficult for you to make?

Write 5 friends with whom you want to share this dish

....

....

....

....

....

INGREDIENTS

- 4 boneless, skinless chicken breasts
- 2 tbsp olive oil
- 2 tbsp lemon juice
- 2 tsp dried oregano
- 1 tsp dried thyme
- 1 tsp garlic powder
- Salt and pepper to taste
- 1 cup uncooked quinoa
- 2 cups low-sodium chicken broth
- 1 cup cherry tomatoes, halved
- 1/4 cup chopped fresh parsley
- 1 avocado, diced

For the Fertility-Boosting Dressing:
- 2 tbsp olive oil
- 1 tbsp lemon juice
- 1 tsp Dijon mustard
- 1 tsp honey
- Salt and pepper to taste

How would you rate this dish?

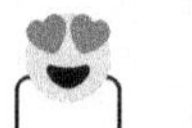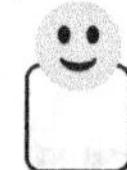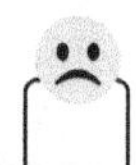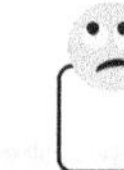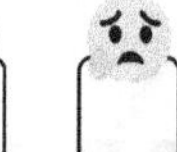

1. Preheat oven to 400°F.

2. In a shallow baking dish, combine the olive oil, lemon juice, oregano, thyme, garlic powder, salt, and pepper. Add the chicken breasts and turn to coat both sides.

3. Bake the chicken for 25-30 minutes, until cooked through.

4. Meanwhile, cook the quinoa: In a medium saucepan, bring the chicken broth to a boil. Add the quinoa, cover, and reduce heat to low. Simmer for 15-20 minutes, until quinoa is tender. Fluff with a fork.

5. In a small bowl, whisk together the ingredients for the fertility-boosting dressing.

6. In a large bowl, combine the cooked quinoa, cherry tomatoes, parsley, and avocado. Drizzle the dressing over the top and toss to coat.

7. Serve the lemon herb chicken breasts over the quinoa salad.

This dish is packed with fertility-boosting nutrients:

- Chicken - a lean protein source
- Quinoa - a complete protein and source of complex carbs
- Avocado - rich in healthy fats that support hormone production
- Tomatoes - contain the antioxidant lycopene
- Lemon, mustard, and honey - provide additional antioxidants

Enjoy this delicious and nutritious meal!

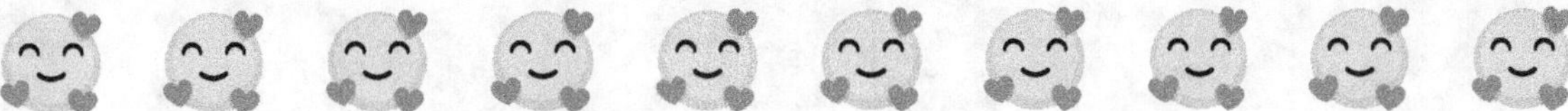

87. Chicken and chickpea stew with tomatoes

 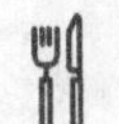

🕐 Prep Time :   🕐 Cook Time :   🍴 Servings :

Is this dish easy or difficult for you to make?

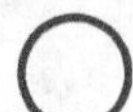 ◯   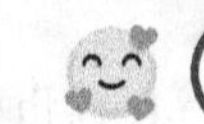 ◯

Write 5 friends with whom you want to share this dish ....

INGREDIENTS

- 1 lb boneless, skinless chicken thighs, cut into 1-inch pieces
- 2 tbsp olive oil
- 1 onion, diced
- 3 cloves garlic, minced
- 1 tsp ground cumin
- 1 tsp paprika
- 1/2 tsp dried oregano
- 1/4 tsp cayenne pepper (optional)
- 1 (15 oz) can diced tomatoes
- 1 (15 oz) can chickpeas, drained and rinsed
- 2 cups low-sodium chicken broth
- 1 cup frozen peas
- Salt and pepper to taste
- Chopped fresh parsley for garnish

1. In a large pot or Dutch oven, heat the olive oil over medium-high heat. Add the chicken and cook for 3-4 minutes, until lightly browned.

2. Add the onion and cook for 5 minutes, until translucent. Stir in the garlic, cumin, paprika, oregano, and cayenne (if using). Cook for 1 minute until fragrant.

3. Pour in the diced tomatoes, chickpeas, and chicken broth. Bring the mixture to a boil, then reduce heat and let simmer for 15-20 minutes, until the chicken is cooked through.

4. Stir in the frozen peas and cook for 5 more minutes. Season with salt and pepper to taste.

5. Serve the stew warm, garnished with chopped fresh parsley.

This dish is packed with fertility-boosting nutrients:

- Chicken - a lean protein source
- Chickpeas - a good source of folate, zinc, and protein
- Tomatoes - rich in the antioxidant lycopene
- Peas - high in folate, which is important for fertility
- Olive oil - provides healthy fats that support hormone production

The combination of these ingredients can help support fertility in both men and women.

Enjoy this delicious and nutritious chicken and chickpea stew!

How would you rate this dish?

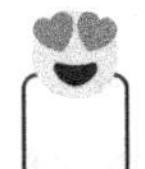 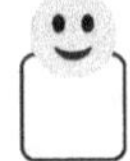  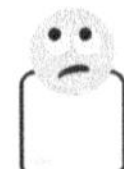 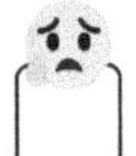

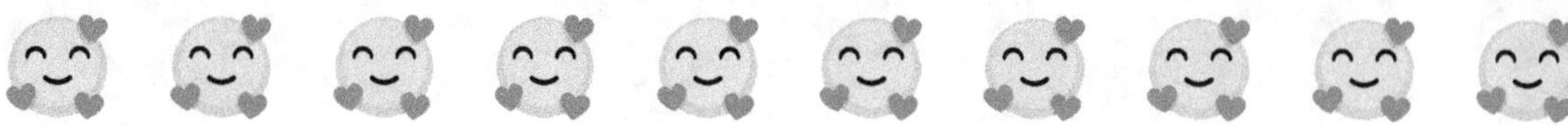

88. BBQ chicken with a side of coleslaw

 *Let's do that and fill in the time here* ✓ Prep Time : 🕐 Cook Time : 🍴 Servings :

Is this dish easy or difficult for you to make?

 😭 ○   🙂 ○

Write 5 friends with whom you want to share this dish
....
....
....
....
....

INGREDIENTS

For the BBQ Chicken:
- 4 boneless, skinless chicken breasts
- 1/2 cup barbecue sauce (look for one without added sugars)
- 1 tbsp olive oil
- 1 tsp smoked paprika
- 1/2 tsp garlic powder
- Salt and pepper to taste

For the Coleslaw:
- 1/2 head green cabbage, shredded
- 1/2 head red cabbage, shredded
- 1 carrot, grated
- 1/2 cup plain Greek yogurt
- 2 tbsp apple cider vinegar
- 1 tsp Dijon mustard
- 1 tsp honey
- Salt and pepper to taste

For the BBQ Chicken:
1. Preheat grill or grill pan to medium-high heat.
2. In a shallow dish, mix together the barbecue sauce, olive oil, smoked paprika, garlic powder, salt, and pepper.
3. Add the chicken breasts and turn to coat both sides.
4. Grill the chicken for 6-8 minutes per side, until cooked through.

For the Coleslaw:
1. In a large bowl, combine the shredded green and red cabbage, and grated carrot.
2. In a small bowl, whisk together the Greek yogurt, apple cider vinegar, Dijon mustard, honey, salt, and pepper.
3. Pour the dressing over the cabbage mixture and toss to coat.

To Serve:
1. Serve the grilled BBQ chicken with the coleslaw on the side.

This meal is packed with fertility-boosting nutrients:

- Chicken - a lean protein source
- Cabbage - high in folate, vitamin C, and antioxidants
- Greek yogurt - provides probiotics and calcium
- Olive oil and avocado oil - healthy fats that support hormone production
- Mustard and apple cider vinegar - contain antioxidants

The combination of these ingredients can help support fertility in both men and women.

Enjoy this delicious and nutritious BBQ chicken and coleslaw!

How would you rate this dish?

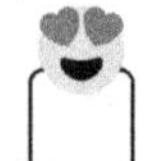 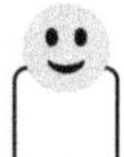 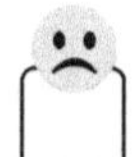 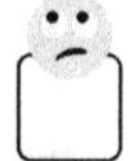 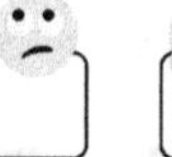 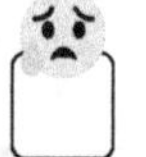

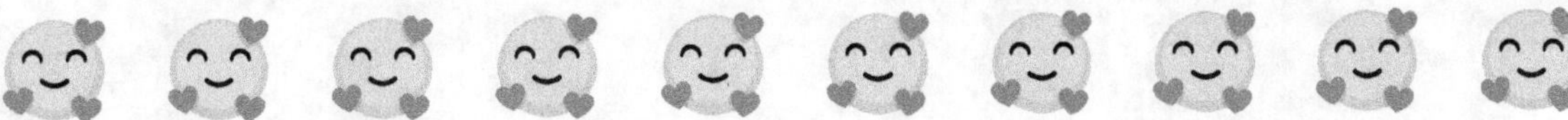

89. Stuffed chicken breast with spinach and feta

 Prep Time :   Cook Time :   Servings :

Is this dish easy or difficult for you to make?

Write 5 friends with whom you want to share this dish
....
....
....
....
....

INGREDIENTS

- 4 boneless, skinless chicken breasts
- 4 oz crumbled feta cheese
- 1 cup fresh spinach, chopped
- 2 cloves garlic, minced
- 1 tbsp olive oil
- 1/4 tsp dried oregano
- Salt and pepper to taste

For the Fertility-Boosting Sauce:
- 1/2 cup plain Greek yogurt
- 2 tbsp lemon juice
- 1 tsp Dijon mustard
- 1 tsp honey
- Salt and pepper to taste

1. Preheat oven to 400°F. Lightly grease a baking dish.

2. In a medium bowl, mix together the feta, spinach, garlic, olive oil, oregano, salt, and pepper.

3. Slice each chicken breast horizontally to create a pocket. Stuff each pocket with the spinach-feta mixture.

4. Place the stuffed chicken breasts in the prepared baking dish. Bake for 25-30 minutes, until the chicken is cooked through.

For the Fertility-Boosting Sauce:
5. In a small bowl, whisk together the Greek yogurt, lemon juice, Dijon mustard, honey, salt, and pepper.

To Serve:
6. Drizzle the fertility-boosting sauce over the top of the stuffed chicken breasts.

This dish is packed with fertility-boosting nutrients:

- Chicken - a lean protein source
- Spinach - high in folate, which is important for fertility
- Feta cheese - provides calcium and protein
- Greek yogurt - rich in probiotics and calcium
- Lemon, mustard, and honey - contain antioxidants

The combination of these ingredients can help support fertility in both men and women.

Enjoy this delicious and nutritious stuffed chicken dish!

How would you rate this dish?

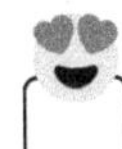 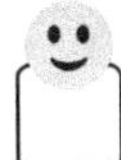 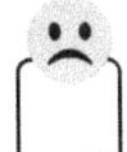 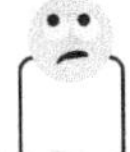 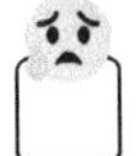

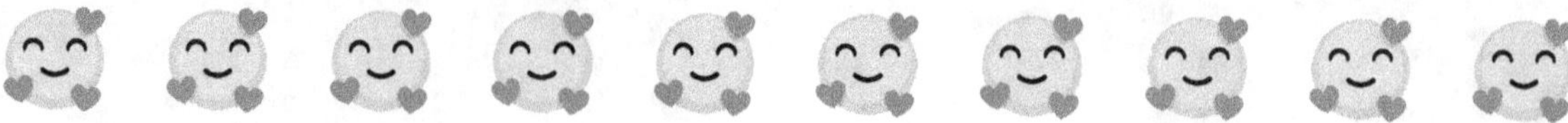

90. Turkey and vegetable kabobs with whole-grain pita

 Prep Time :   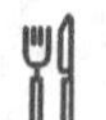 Cook Time :   Servings :

Is this dish easy or difficult for you to make?

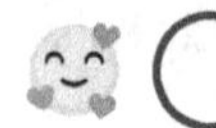 ◯   ◯

Write 5 friends with whom you want to share this dish

....

....

....

....

....

INGREDIENTS

- 1 lb ground turkey
- 1 zucchini, cut into 1-inch pieces
- 1 red bell pepper, cut into 1-inch pieces
- 1 red onion, cut into 1-inch pieces
- 8 cherry tomatoes
- 2 tbsp olive oil
- 1 tsp dried oregano
- 1/2 tsp garlic powder
- Salt and pepper to taste
- 4 whole-grain pita breads, warmed

For the Fertility-Boosting Tzatziki Sauce:
- 1 cup plain Greek yogurt
- 1 cucumber, grated and squeezed dry
- 2 tbsp lemon juice
- 1 clove garlic, minced
- 1 tbsp chopped fresh dill
- Salt and pepper to taste

1. Preheat grill or grill pan to medium-high heat.

2. In a large bowl, mix together the ground turkey, zucchini, bell pepper, onion, and tomatoes. Drizzle with the olive oil and sprinkle with the oregano, garlic powder, salt, and pepper. Toss to coat.

3. Thread the turkey and vegetable pieces onto skewers.

4. Grill the kabobs for 12-15 minutes, turning occasionally, until the turkey is cooked through and the vegetables are tender.

For the Tzatziki Sauce:
5. In a medium bowl, combine the Greek yogurt, grated cucumber, lemon juice, garlic, and dill. Season with salt and pepper.

To Serve:
6. Serve the grilled turkey and vegetable kabobs with the warm whole-grain pita breads and the fertility-boosting tzatziki sauce.

This dish is packed with fertility-boosting nutrients:

- Turkey - a lean protein source
- Vegetables (zucchini, bell pepper, onion, tomatoes) - high in antioxidants and vitamins
- Greek yogurt - rich in probiotics and calcium
- Lemon and dill - contain antioxidants

The whole-grain pita provides complex carbs for sustained energy.

Enjoy this delicious and nutritious grilled kabob meal!

How would you rate this dish?

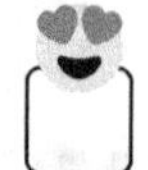 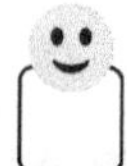 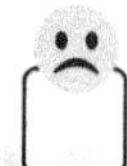  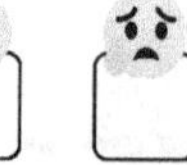

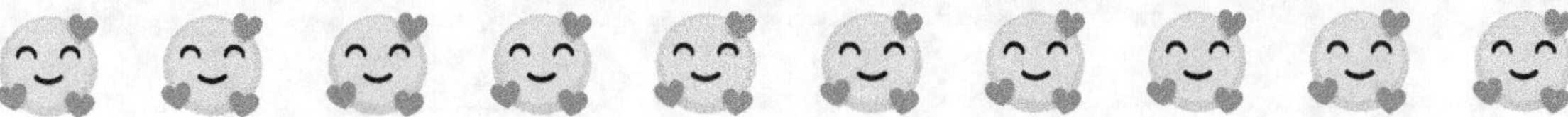

91. Wild rice pilaf with cranberries and almonds

Prep Time :   Cook Time :   Servings :

Is this dish easy or difficult for you to make?

 ○    ○

Write 5 ....
friends
with ....
whom
you ....
want to
share ....
this
dish ....

INGREDIENTS

- 1 cup uncooked wild rice
- 2 cups low-sodium chicken or vegetable broth
- 1/2 cup dried cranberries
- 1/4 cup sliced almonds
- 2 tbsp olive oil
- 1 onion, diced
- 2 cloves garlic, minced
- 1 tsp dried thyme
- Salt and pepper to taste
- Chopped fresh parsley for garnish

1. In a medium saucepan, bring the wild rice and broth to a boil. Reduce heat, cover and simmer for 45-50 minutes, until rice is tender. Fluff with a fork.

2. In a large skillet, heat the olive oil over medium heat. Add the diced onion and sauté for 5-7 minutes until translucent.

3. Stir in the minced garlic and dried thyme. Cook for 1 minute until fragrant.

4. Add the cooked wild rice, dried cranberries, and sliced almonds to the skillet. Toss everything together and cook for 2-3 minutes to allow the flavors to meld.

5. Season the pilaf with salt and pepper to taste.

6. Transfer the wild rice pilaf to a serving bowl and garnish with chopped fresh parsley.

This dish is packed with fertility-boosting nutrients:

- Wild rice - a whole grain that's high in fiber, protein, and antioxidants
- Cranberries - rich in antioxidants that may help improve sperm quality
- Almonds - a good source of zinc, which is important for male fertility
- Olive oil - provides healthy fats that support hormone production
- Garlic - contains allicin, which may improve sperm quality

The combination of these ingredients can help support fertility in both men and women.

Enjoy this delicious and nutritious wild rice pilaf!

How would you rate this dish?

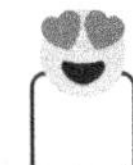 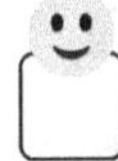 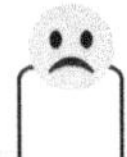 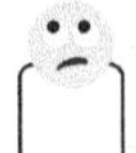 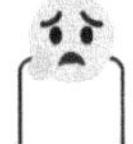

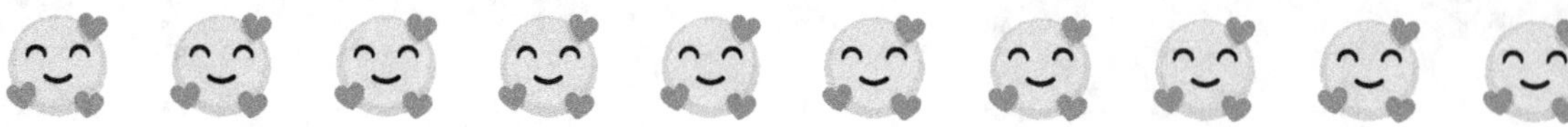

92. Barley risotto with mushrooms and peas

Prep Time :   Cook Time :   Servings :

Is this dish easy or difficult for you to make?

 ◯    ◯

Write 5 friends with whom you want to share this dish ....

INGREDIENTS

- 1 cup pearl barley
- 4 cups low-sodium vegetable or chicken broth
- 1 tbsp olive oil
- 8 oz cremini mushrooms, sliced
- 1 onion, diced
- 3 cloves garlic, minced
- 1 cup frozen peas
- 1/4 cup grated Parmesan cheese
- 2 tbsp chopped fresh parsley
- Salt and pepper to taste

1. In a medium saucepan, bring the barley and broth to a boil. Reduce heat, cover and simmer for 25-30 minutes, until barley is tender. Drain any excess liquid.

2. In a large skillet, heat the olive oil over medium heat. Add the sliced mushrooms and cook for 5-7 minutes, until browned.

3. Add the diced onion to the skillet and cook for 3-4 minutes until translucent. Stir in the minced garlic and cook for 1 minute.

4. Add the cooked barley to the skillet with the mushrooms and onions. Stir to combine.

5. Stir in the frozen peas and cook for 2-3 minutes until heated through.

6. Remove from heat and stir in the grated Parmesan cheese. Season with salt and pepper to taste.

7. Garnish the barley risotto with chopped fresh parsley before serving.

This dish is packed with fertility-boosting nutrients:

- Barley - a whole grain that's high in fiber, protein, and antioxidants
- Mushrooms - contain selenium, which is important for sperm health
- Peas - high in folate, which is crucial for fertility in both men and women
- Parmesan cheese - provides calcium and protein
- Olive oil - a source of healthy fats that support hormone production

The combination of these ingredients can help support fertility in couples.

How would you rate this dish?

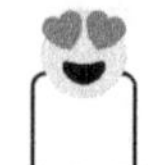 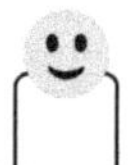  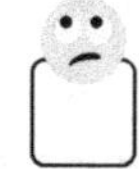 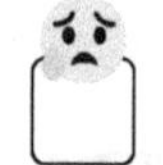

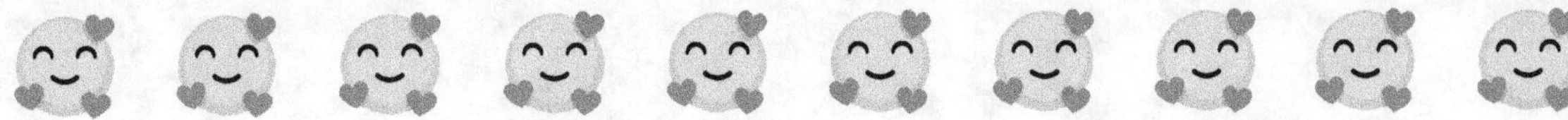

93. Quinoa and black bean bowl with cilantro lime dressing

Let's do that and fill in the time here   Prep Time :   Cook Time :   Servings :

Is this dish easy or difficult for you to make?

 ○   ○

Write 5 friends with whom you want to share this dish ....

INGREDIENTS

For the Bowl:
- 1 cup uncooked quinoa, rinsed
- 1 (15 oz) can black beans, drained and rinsed
- 1 cup cherry tomatoes, halved
- 1 avocado, diced
- 1/2 cup corn kernels (fresh or frozen)
- 1/4 cup chopped fresh cilantro

For the Cilantro Lime Dressing:
- 1/4 cup olive oil
- 2 tbsp lime juice
- 2 tbsp chopped fresh cilantro
- 1 clove garlic, minced
- 1 tsp Dijon mustard
- 1 tsp honey
- Salt and pepper to taste

1. Cook the quinoa according to package instructions. Fluff with a fork and set aside.

2. In a large bowl, combine the cooked quinoa, black beans, cherry tomatoes, avocado, corn, and chopped cilantro.

For the Cilantro Lime Dressing:
3. In a small bowl, whisk together the olive oil, lime juice, cilantro, garlic, Dijon mustard, and honey. Season with salt and pepper.

4. Drizzle the cilantro lime dressing over the quinoa and black bean bowl. Toss gently to coat.

5. Serve immediately, garnished with extra chopped cilantro if desired.

This dish is packed with fertility-boosting nutrients:

- Quinoa - a complete protein and source of complex carbs
- Black beans - high in folate, zinc, and protein
- Avocado - rich in healthy fats that support hormone production
- Tomatoes - contain the antioxidant lycopene
- Cilantro and lime - provide additional antioxidants

The combination of these ingredients can help support fertility in both men and women.

Enjoy this delicious and nutritious quinoa and black bean bowl!

How would you rate this dish?

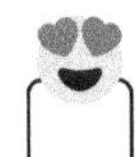 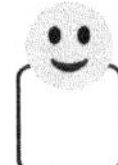 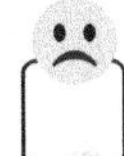 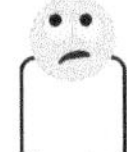 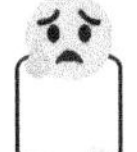

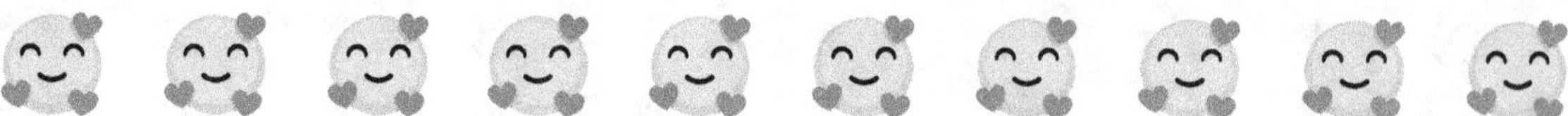

94. Bulgur wheat salad with pomegranate and mint

Prep Time :   Cook Time :   Servings :

Is this dish easy or difficult for you to make?

 ○   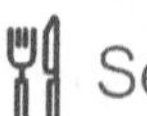 ○

Write 5 ....
friends
with   ....
whom
you   ....
want to
share   ....
this
dish   ....

INGREDIENTS

- 1 cup uncooked bulgur wheat
- 1 1/2 cups boiling water
- 1 cup pomegranate arils
- 1 cucumber, diced
- 1/2 cup chopped fresh mint
- 1/4 cup chopped fresh parsley
- 2 tbsp olive oil
- 2 tbsp lemon juice
- 1 tsp Dijon mustard
- 1 tsp honey
- Salt and pepper to taste

1. In a medium bowl, combine the uncooked bulgur wheat and boiling water. Cover and let sit for 15-20 minutes, until the bulgur is tender and the water is absorbed. Fluff with a fork.

2. In a large bowl, combine the cooked bulgur, pomegranate arils, diced cucumber, chopped mint, and chopped parsley.

For the Dressing:
3. In a small bowl, whisk together the olive oil, lemon juice, Dijon mustard, and honey. Season with salt and pepper.

4. Pour the dressing over the bulgur salad and toss gently to coat.

5. Serve the bulgur wheat salad chilled or at room temperature.

This dish is packed with fertility-boosting nutrients:

- Bulgur wheat - a whole grain that's high in fiber, protein, and antioxidants
- Pomegranate - rich in antioxidants that may help improve sperm quality
- Mint and parsley - provide additional antioxidants
- Olive oil - a source of healthy fats that support hormone production
- Lemon and Dijon mustard - contain additional antioxidants

The combination of these ingredients can help support fertility in both men and women.

Enjoy this delicious and nutritious bulgur wheat salad!

How would you rate this dish?

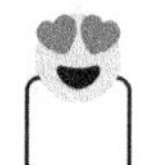 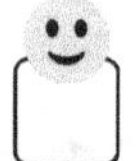 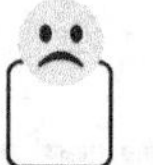 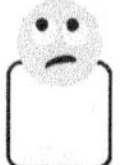 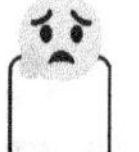

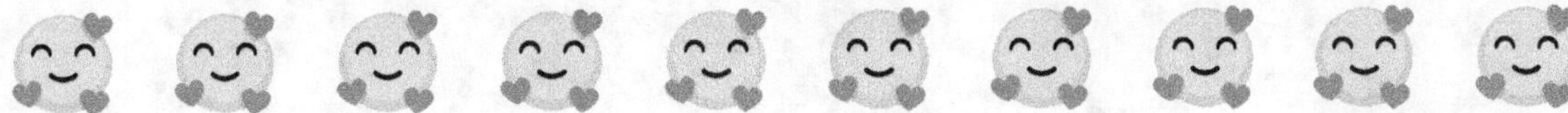

95. Farro and roasted vegetable bowl with tahini dressing

 Prep Time :   Cook Time :   Servings :

Is this dish easy or difficult for you to make?

 ◯   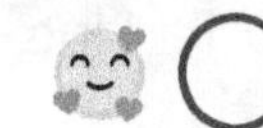 ◯

Write 5 ....
friends
with ....
whom
you ....
want to
share ....
this
dish ....

INGREDIENTS

For the Roasted Vegetables:
- 1 lb sweet potatoes, cubed
- 1 red bell pepper, chopped
- 1 zucchini, chopped
- 1 red onion, sliced
- 2 tbsp olive oil
- Salt and pepper to taste

For the Farro:
- 1 cup uncooked farro
- 3 cups low-sodium vegetable or chicken broth

For the Tahini Dressing:
- 1/4 cup tahini
- 2 tbsp lemon juice
- 1 tbsp honey
- 1 garlic clove, minced
- 2-3 tbsp water, to thin
- Salt and pepper to taste

To Serve:
- 1/2 cup cooked chickpeas
- 2 tbsp toasted sesame seeds
- Chopped fresh parsley

How would you rate this dish?

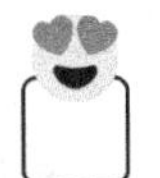 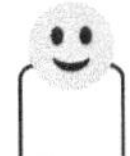 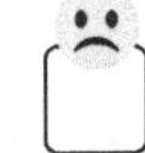 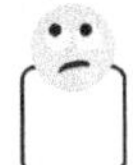 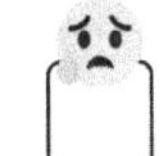

1. Preheat oven to 400°F. Toss the cubed sweet potatoes, bell pepper, zucchini, and onion with the olive oil on a baking sheet. Season with salt and pepper. Roast for 25-30 minutes, until vegetables are tender.

2. Meanwhile, cook the farro: In a medium saucepan, bring the farro and broth to a boil. Reduce heat, cover and simmer for 20-25 minutes, until farro is tender. Drain any excess liquid.

3. In a small bowl, whisk together the tahini, lemon juice, honey, garlic, and 2-3 tbsp water to thin the dressing to your desired consistency. Season with salt and pepper.

4. In a large bowl, combine the roasted vegetables, cooked farro, chickpeas, and tahini dressing. Toss to coat.

5. Serve the farro and vegetable bowl garnished with toasted sesame seeds and chopped fresh parsley.

This dish is packed with fertility-boosting nutrients:

- Farro - a whole grain that's high in fiber, protein, and antioxidants
- Sweet potatoes - rich in vitamin A, which is important for fertility
- Bell peppers and zucchini - high in vitamin C and other antioxidants
- Tahini - a good source of zinc, which supports male fertility
- Chickpeas - high in folate, which is crucial for fertility in both men and women

The combination of these ingredients can help support fertility in couples.

Enjoy this delicious and nutritious farro and roasted vegetable bowl!

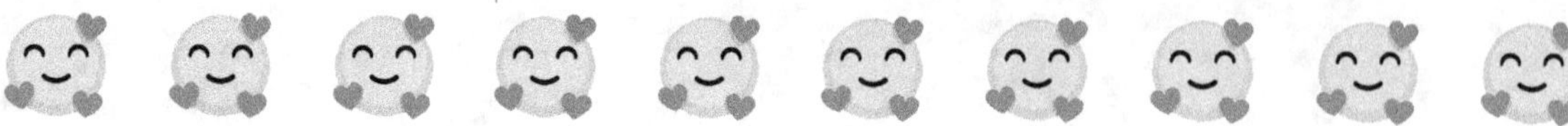

96. Millet with roasted tomatoes and basil

 Prep Time :   Cook Time :   Servings :

Is this dish easy or difficult for you to make?

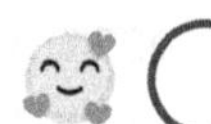 ◯   ◯

Write 5 friends with whom you want to share this dish ....

INGREDIENTS

- 1 cup uncooked millet
- 2 cups low-sodium vegetable or chicken broth
- 1 lb cherry or grape tomatoes, halved
- 2 tbsp olive oil
- 2 cloves garlic, minced
- 1/4 tsp red pepper flakes (optional)
- Salt and pepper to taste
- 1/4 cup chopped fresh basil
- 2 tbsp toasted pine nuts (optional)

1. Preheat oven to 400°F. Line a baking sheet with parchment paper.

2. In a medium saucepan, bring the millet and broth to a boil. Reduce heat, cover and simmer for 20-25 minutes, until millet is tender. Fluff with a fork.

3. Spread the halved tomatoes on the prepared baking sheet. Drizzle with 1 tbsp of the olive oil and season with salt and pepper.

4. Roast the tomatoes for 15-20 minutes, until softened and slightly charred.

5. In a large skillet, heat the remaining 1 tbsp of olive oil over medium heat. Add the minced garlic and red pepper flakes (if using). Cook for 1 minute until fragrant.

6. Add the cooked millet to the skillet and toss to coat in the garlic oil.

7. Stir in the roasted tomatoes and chopped fresh basil. Season with additional salt and pepper to taste.

8. Serve the millet topped with the toasted pine nuts, if desired.

This dish is packed with fertility-boosting nutrients:

- Millet - a gluten-free whole grain that's high in protein, fiber, and antioxidants
- Tomatoes - rich in the antioxidant lycopene, which may help improve sperm quality
- Basil - provides additional antioxidants
- Olive oil - a source of healthy fats that support hormone production
- Pine nuts - contain zinc, which is important for male fertility

How would you rate this dish?

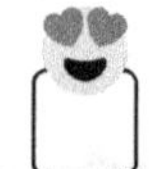 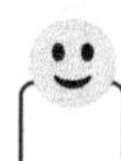 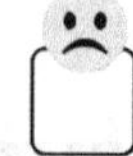 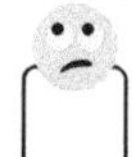 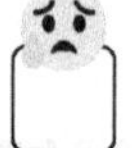

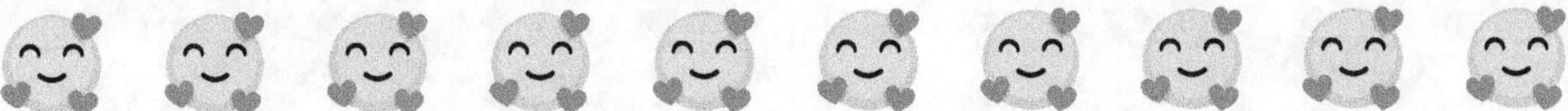

97. Brown rice stir-fry with tofu and vegetables

Prep Time :   Cook Time :   Servings :

Is this dish easy or difficult for you to make?

 ◯    ◯

Write 5 friends with whom you want to share this dish

....
....
....
....
....

INGREDIENTS

- 1 cup uncooked brown rice
- 1 block extra-firm tofu, cubed
- 2 tbsp sesame oil, divided
- 1 red bell pepper, sliced
- 1 cup broccoli florets
- 1 cup sliced mushrooms
- 1 cup snow peas
- 3 cloves garlic, minced
- 1 tbsp grated fresh ginger
- 2 tbsp low-sodium soy sauce
- 1 tbsp rice vinegar
- 1 tsp honey
- Salt and pepper to taste
- Chopped green onions and sesame seeds for garnish

1. Cook the brown rice according to package instructions. Set aside.

2. In a large skillet or wok, heat 1 tbsp of the sesame oil over medium-high heat. Add the cubed tofu and cook for 5-7 minutes, turning occasionally, until lightly browned on all sides. Remove tofu from pan and set aside.

3. Add the remaining 1 tbsp sesame oil to the pan. Stir-fry the bell pepper, broccoli, mushrooms, and snow peas for 5-7 minutes, until tender-crisp.

4. Add the garlic and ginger to the pan and cook for 1 minute until fragrant.

5. Return the cooked tofu to the pan. Stir in the soy sauce, rice vinegar, and honey. Toss to coat everything evenly.

6. Add the cooked brown rice to the stir-fry and gently mix everything together.

7. Season with salt and pepper to taste.

8. Serve the brown rice stir-fry warm, garnished with chopped green onions and sesame seeds.

This dish is packed with fertility-boosting nutrients:

- Brown rice - a whole grain that's high in fiber and antioxidants
- Tofu - a plant-based protein source that's rich in isoflavones
- Vegetables (bell pepper, broccoli, mushrooms, snow peas) - high in vitamins, minerals, and antioxidants
- Sesame oil and sesame seeds - contain zinc, which is important for male fertility
- Ginger and garlic - provide additional antioxidants

How would you rate this dish?

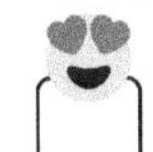 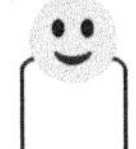 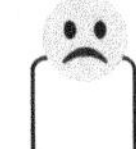 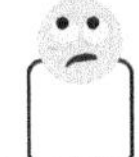 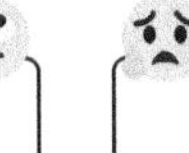

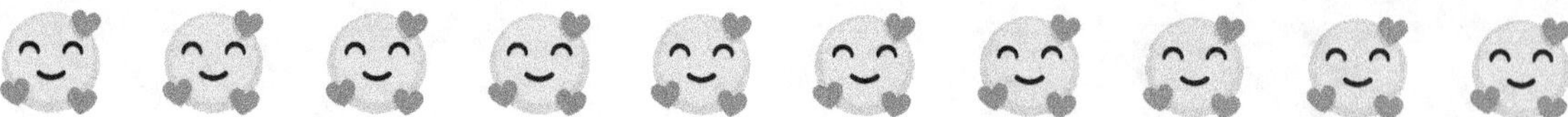

98. Couscous with grilled vegetables and chickpeas

 Prep Time :   Cook Time :   Servings :

Is this dish easy or difficult for you to make?

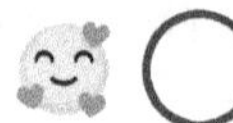 ◯   ◯

Write 5 ....
friends
with ....
whom
you ....
want to
share ....
this
dish ....

INGREDIENTS

- 1 cup uncooked whole wheat couscous
- 1 1/4 cups low-sodium vegetable or chicken broth
- 1 zucchini, sliced into rounds
- 1 red bell pepper, sliced
- 1 red onion, sliced into rings
- 1 (15 oz) can chickpeas, drained and rinsed
- 2 tbsp olive oil, divided
- 1 tbsp lemon juice
- 2 tsp Dijon mustard
- 1 tsp honey
- 1/4 cup chopped fresh parsley
- Salt and pepper to taste

1. Prepare the couscous according to package instructions, using the vegetable or chicken broth instead of water. Fluff with a fork and set aside.

2. Preheat grill or grill pan to medium-high heat. Toss the zucchini, bell pepper, and onion slices with 1 tbsp of the olive oil. Season with salt and pepper.

3. Grill the vegetables for 5-7 minutes per side, until tender and charred in spots. Remove from grill and let cool slightly, then chop into bite-sized pieces.

4. In a large bowl, combine the grilled vegetables, chickpeas, and cooked couscous.

5. In a small bowl, whisk together the remaining 1 tbsp olive oil, lemon juice, Dijon mustard, and honey. Season with salt and pepper.

6. Pour the dressing over the couscous and vegetable mixture. Toss gently to coat.

7. Stir in the chopped fresh parsley.

8. Serve the couscous salad warm or at room temperature.

This dish is packed with fertility-boosting nutrients:

- Whole wheat couscous - a source of complex carbs and fiber
- Vegetables (zucchini, bell pepper, onion) - high in antioxidants
- Chickpeas - a good source of protein, folate, and zinc
- Olive oil - provides healthy fats that support hormone production
- Lemon, mustard, and honey - contain additional antioxidants

How would you rate this dish?

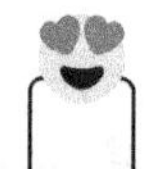 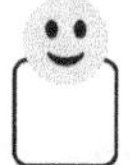 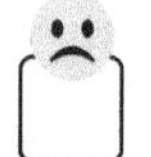 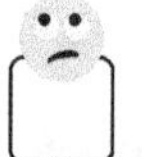 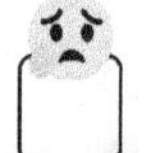

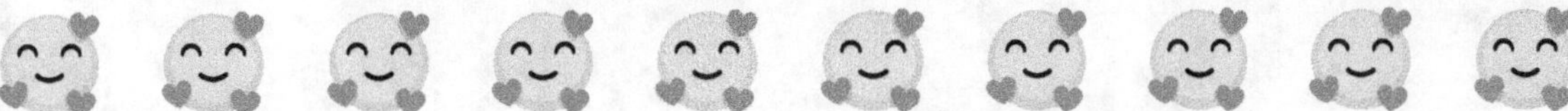

99. Polenta with sautéed spinach and mushrooms

🕐 Prep Time :   🕐 Cook Time :   🍴 Servings :

Is this dish easy or difficult for you to make?

 ⬡   ⬡

Write 5 friends with whom you want to share this dish ....

INGREDIENTS

- 1 cup dry polenta
- 4 cups low-sodium vegetable or chicken broth
- 1 tbsp olive oil
- 8 oz cremini mushrooms, sliced
- 3 cloves garlic, minced
- 5 oz baby spinach
- 2 tbsp grated Parmesan cheese
- Salt and pepper to taste

For the Fertility-Boosting Sauce:
- 1/4 cup plain Greek yogurt
- 2 tbsp lemon juice
- 1 tsp Dijon mustard
- 1 tsp honey
- Salt and pepper to taste

How would you rate this dish?

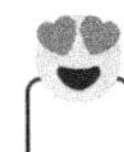 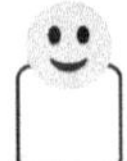 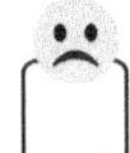 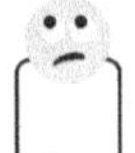 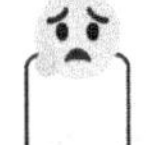

1. Bring the broth to a boil in a medium saucepan. Slowly whisk in the polenta. Reduce heat to low and cook, stirring frequently, for 15-20 minutes until thickened. Season with salt and pepper.

2. In a large skillet, heat the olive oil over medium-high heat. Add the sliced mushrooms and cook for 5-7 minutes, until browned.

3. Add the minced garlic to the skillet and cook for 1 minute until fragrant.

4. Stir in the baby spinach and cook for 2-3 minutes, until wilted.

5. In a small bowl, whisk together the ingredients for the fertility-boosting sauce.

6. Spoon the cooked polenta into bowls. Top with the sautéed spinach and mushrooms. Drizzle the fertility-boosting sauce over the top.

7. Sprinkle with the grated Parmesan cheese before serving.

This dish is packed with fertility-boosting nutrients:

- Polenta - a gluten-free whole grain that's high in fiber and antioxidants
- Spinach - rich in folate, which is crucial for fertility
- Mushrooms - contain selenium, which supports sperm health
- Greek yogurt - provides probiotics and calcium
- Lemon, mustard, and honey - contain additional antioxidants
- Parmesan cheese - a source of calcium

The combination of these ingredients can help support fertility in both men and women.

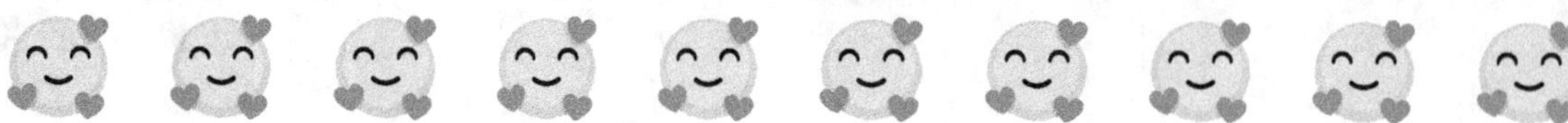

100. Wild rice and lentil casserole with herbs

 *Let's do that and fill in the time here* Prep Time :    Cook Time :   Servings :

Is this dish easy or difficult for you to make?

 ◯   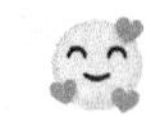 ◯

Write 5 friends with whom you want to share this dish ....

INGREDIENTS

- 1 cup uncooked wild rice
- 1 cup uncooked brown lentils
- 4 cups low-sodium vegetable or chicken broth
- 1 onion, diced
- 3 cloves garlic, minced
- 2 carrots, peeled and diced
- 2 celery stalks, diced
- 1 cup sliced mushrooms
- 1/4 cup chopped fresh parsley
- 2 tbsp chopped fresh thyme
- 1 tsp dried oregano
- Salt and pepper to taste
- 1/4 cup grated Parmesan cheese (optional)

1. Preheat oven to 375°F. Grease a 9x13 inch baking dish.

2. In a large saucepan, combine the wild rice, lentils, and broth. Bring to a boil, then reduce heat, cover and simmer for 30-35 minutes, until rice and lentils are tender. Drain any excess liquid.

3. In a large skillet, sauté the onion and garlic in a bit of olive oil over medium heat for 3-4 minutes until translucent.

4. Add the diced carrots, celery, and sliced mushrooms to the skillet. Cook for 5-7 minutes, until vegetables are tender.

5. Transfer the cooked wild rice and lentils to the prepared baking dish. Stir in the sautéed vegetables, chopped parsley, thyme, and oregano. Season with salt and pepper.

6. If using, sprinkle the grated Parmesan cheese over the top of the casserole.

7. Bake for 20-25 minutes, until heated through and the cheese is melted.

This dish is packed with fertility-boosting nutrients:

- Wild rice - a whole grain that's high in fiber, protein, and antioxidants
- Lentils - a good source of folate, iron, and zinc
- Vegetables (carrots, celery, mushrooms) - rich in vitamins and minerals
- Herbs (parsley, thyme, oregano) - provide additional antioxidants
- Parmesan cheese - a source of calcium

How would you rate this dish?

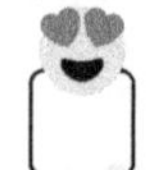 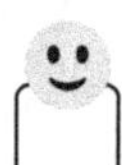 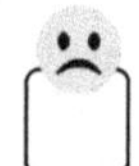 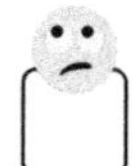 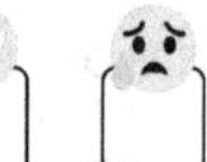

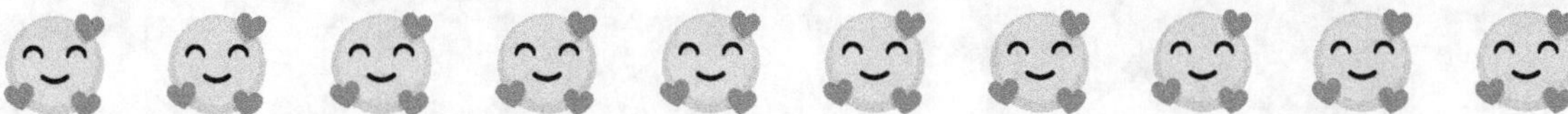

101. Berry parfait with Greek yogurt and honey

Let's do that and fill in the time here

🕐 Prep Time :   🕐 Cook Time :   🍴 Servings :

Is this dish easy or difficult for you to make?

 ◯   😊 ◯

Write 5 friends with whom you want to share this dish

....
....
....
....
....

INGREDIENTS

- 2 cups plain Greek yogurt
- 1/4 cup honey
- 1 tsp vanilla extract
- 2 cups mixed berries (such as strawberries, blueberries, raspberries)
- 1/4 cup chopped walnuts or almonds

1. In a medium bowl, mix together the Greek yogurt, honey, and vanilla extract until well combined.

2. In parfait glasses or small bowls, layer the yogurt mixture and the mixed berries, starting and ending with the yogurt.

3. Top each parfait with a sprinkle of the chopped nuts.

4. Refrigerate the parfaits for at least 30 minutes before serving to allow the flavors to meld.

This berry parfait is packed with fertility-boosting nutrients:

- Greek yogurt - provides probiotics, calcium, and protein
- Honey - contains antioxidants that may help improve sperm quality
- Berries - rich in antioxidants and vitamins that support fertility
- Nuts - a good source of zinc, which is important for male fertility

The combination of these ingredients can help support fertility in both men and women.

Some additional tips:

- Use a variety of berries for maximum nutrient benefits.
- Substitute other nuts like almonds or pecans if you prefer.
- Drizzle a bit of extra honey over the top, if desired.

Enjoy this delicious and nutritious berry parfait!

How would you rate this dish?

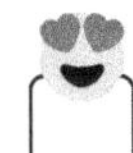 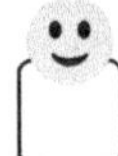  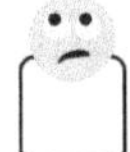 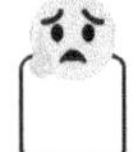

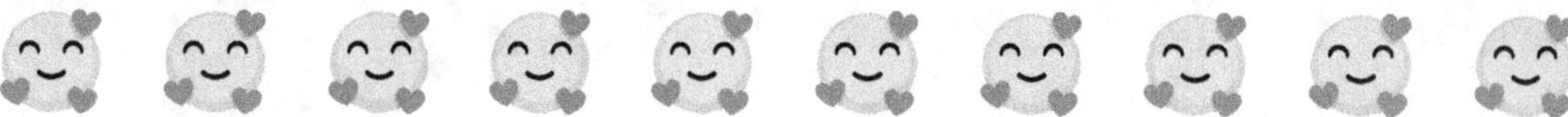

102. Baked apples with cinnamon and walnuts

Let's do that and fill in the time here  Prep Time :   Cook Time :    Servings :

Is this dish easy or difficult for you to make?

Write 5 friends with whom you want to share this dish ....

INGREDIENTS

- 4 medium-sized apples (such as Honeycrisp or Gala)
- 1/4 cup chopped walnuts
- 2 tbsp honey
- 1 tsp ground cinnamon
- 1/4 tsp ground nutmeg
- 2 tbsp water

1. Preheat oven to 375°F. Lightly grease a baking dish.

2. Core the apples, leaving the bottom intact so they can stand upright. Place the apples in the prepared baking dish.

3. In a small bowl, mix together the chopped walnuts, honey, cinnamon, and nutmeg.

4. Spoon the walnut-cinnamon mixture into the center of each apple, packing it in gently.

5. Pour the water into the bottom of the baking dish.

6. Bake the apples for 30-35 minutes, until they are tender when pierced with a fork.

7. Serve the baked apples warm, with the juices from the baking dish spooned over the top.

This dessert is packed with fertility-boosting nutrients:

- Apples - contain antioxidants that may help improve sperm quality
- Walnuts - a good source of omega-3 fatty acids and zinc, which support male fertility
- Cinnamon - contains antioxidants that may help regulate hormones
- Honey - provides antioxidants that can benefit both male and female fertility

The combination of these ingredients can help support fertility in couples.

You can also try adding a dollop of plain Greek yogurt or a drizzle of almond milk to the baked apples for an extra fertility boost.

Enjoy this delicious and nutritious dessert!

How would you rate this dish?

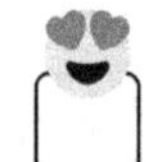 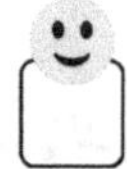  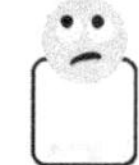 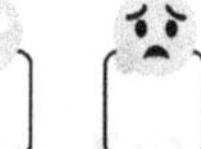

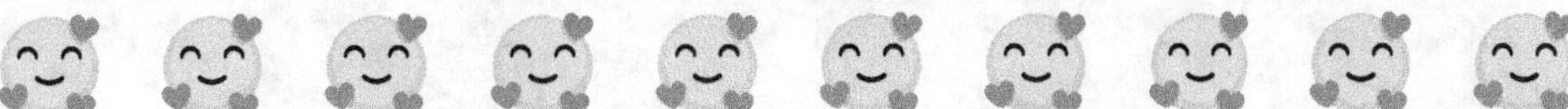

103. Dark chocolate-dipped strawberries

 Prep Time :   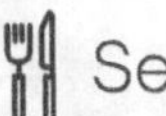 Cook Time :   Servings :

Is this dish easy or difficult for you to make?

○   ○

Write 5 friends with whom you want to share this dish

....

....

....

....

....

INGREDIENTS

- 12 fresh strawberries, washed and patted dry
- 4 oz dark chocolate, chopped (at least 70% cacao)
- 1 tbsp coconut oil

1. Line a baking sheet with parchment paper.

2. In a double boiler or microwave-safe bowl, melt the dark chocolate and coconut oil together, stirring frequently until smooth.

3. Holding them by the stem, dip each strawberry into the melted chocolate, coating about 3/4 of the berry.

4. Gently tap off any excess chocolate and place the dipped strawberries on the prepared baking sheet.

5. Refrigerate the chocolate-dipped strawberries for at least 30 minutes, until the chocolate has hardened.

This simple dessert is packed with fertility-boosting nutrients:

- Strawberries - rich in vitamin C, which is important for fertility in both men and women
- Dark chocolate - contains flavonoids that may help improve sperm quality and motility
- Coconut oil - provides healthy fats that support hormone production

The combination of these ingredients can help support fertility in couples.

Some additional tips:

- Use the highest quality dark chocolate you can find, with at least 70% cacao.
- You can also sprinkle a bit of chopped nuts or drizzle a touch of honey over the dipped strawberries for extra nutrients.
- Store the chocolate-dipped strawberries in the refrigerator until ready to serve.

How would you rate this dish?

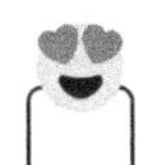 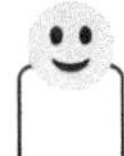  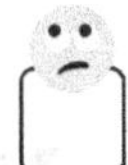 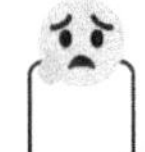

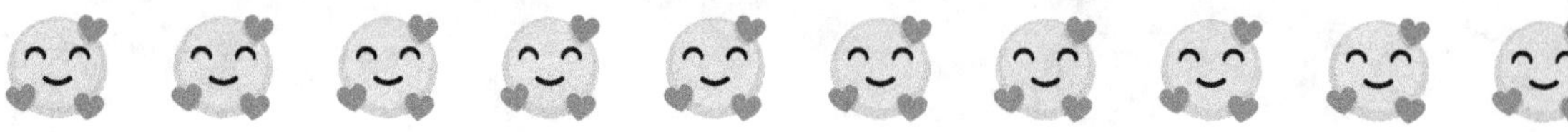

104. Chia seed pudding with mango puree

Prep Time :

Cook Time :

Servings :

Is this dish easy or difficult for you to make?

 ○   ○

Write 5 ....
friends
with ....
whom
you ....
want to
share ....
this
dish ....

INGREDIENTS

For the Chia Seed Pudding:
- 1/4 cup chia seeds
- 1 1/2 cups unsweetened almond milk
- 2 tbsp honey
- 1 tsp vanilla extract

For the Mango Puree:
- 1 ripe mango, peeled and diced
- 1 tbsp honey
- 1 tbsp freshly squeezed lemon juice

For the Chia Seed Pudding:
1. In a medium bowl, whisk together the chia seeds, almond milk, honey, and vanilla extract until well combined.
2. Cover and refrigerate for at least 4 hours, or overnight, stirring occasionally, until thickened.

For the Mango Puree:
1. In a blender or food processor, blend the diced mango, honey, and lemon juice until smooth.

To Assemble:
1. Divide the chia seed pudding evenly between 4 serving bowls or glasses.
2. Top each portion with a generous spoonful of the mango puree.
3. Garnish with extra mango slices, if desired.

This chia seed pudding with mango puree is packed with fertility-boosting nutrients:

- Chia seeds - a great source of omega-3 fatty acids, which support reproductive health
- Mango - rich in vitamin C, an important nutrient for fertility in both men and women
- Almond milk - provides healthy fats that support hormone production
- Honey - contains antioxidants that may help improve sperm quality
- Lemon - provides additional antioxidants

The combination of these ingredients can help support fertility in couples.

Enjoy this delicious and nutritious chia seed pudding!

How would you rate this dish?

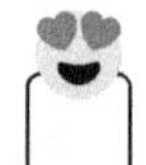 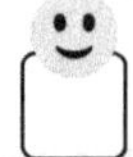 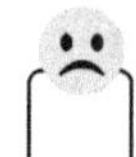 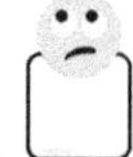 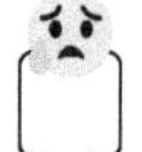

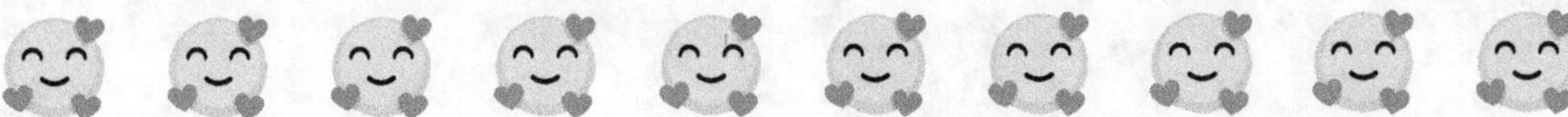

105. Oatmeal cookies with raisins and walnuts

 Prep Time :   Cook Time :   Servings :

Is this dish easy or difficult for you to make?

 ◯   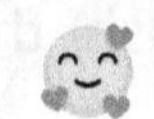 ◯

Write 5 friends with whom you want to share this dish

....

....

....

....

INGREDIENTS

- 1 cup whole wheat flour
- 1 tsp baking soda
- 1/2 tsp ground cinnamon
- 1/4 tsp salt
- 1/2 cup unsalted butter, softened
- 3/4 cup brown sugar
- 1 egg
- 1 tsp vanilla extract
- 1 1/2 cups old-fashioned oats
- 1/2 cup raisins
- 1/2 cup chopped walnuts

How would you rate this dish?

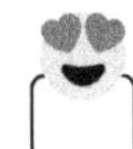 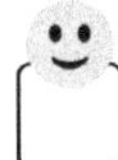  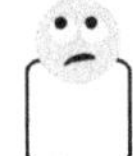 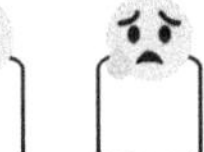

1. Preheat oven to 350°F. Line a baking sheet with parchment paper.

2. In a medium bowl, whisk together the whole wheat flour, baking soda, cinnamon, and salt.

3. In a large bowl, beat the softened butter and brown sugar together until light and fluffy. Beat in the egg and vanilla.

4. Gradually stir the dry ingredients into the wet ingredients until just combined. Fold in the oats, raisins, and chopped walnuts.

5. Scoop rounded tablespoons of dough onto the prepared baking sheet, spacing them about 2 inches apart.

6. Bake for 10-12 minutes, until the cookies are lightly golden around the edges.

7. Allow the cookies to cool on the baking sheet for 5 minutes before transferring to a wire rack to cool completely.

These oatmeal cookies are packed with fertility-boosting nutrients:

- Whole wheat flour - provides complex carbs and fiber
- Oats - a good source of zinc, which supports male fertility
- Raisins - contain antioxidants that may help improve sperm quality
- Walnuts - rich in omega-3 fatty acids that support reproductive health

The combination of these ingredients can help support fertility in both men and women.

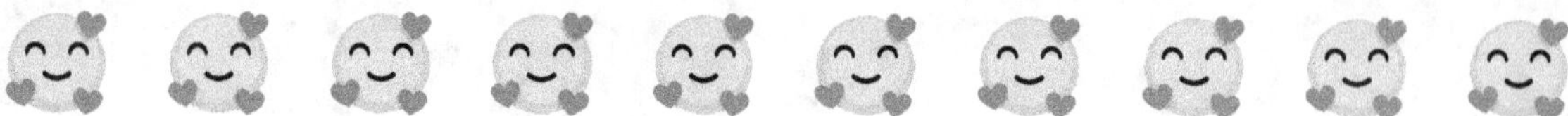

106. Banana and almond butter bites

 Prep Time :    Cook Time :   Servings :

Is this dish easy or difficult for you to make?

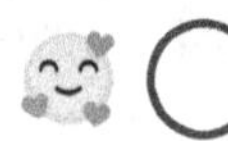 ◯   ◯

Write 5 friends with whom you want to share this dish

....
....
....
....
....

INGREDIENTS

- 2 ripe bananas, mashed
- 1/2 cup creamy almond butter
- 1/4 cup rolled oats
- 2 tablespoons honey (or maple syrup)
- 1/4 teaspoon ground cinnamon
- Pinch of salt

1. In a medium bowl, mash the ripe bananas until smooth.

2. Add the almond butter, rolled oats, honey (or maple syrup), cinnamon, and a pinch of salt. Stir until well combined.

3. Scoop the mixture by the tablespoonful and roll into bite-sized balls. Place the balls on a parchment-lined baking sheet.

4. Refrigerate the bites for at least 30 minutes to allow them to firm up.

5. Serve chilled. Store any leftover bites in an airtight container in the refrigerator for up to 1 week.

These Banana and Almond Butter Bites make a healthy, protein-packed snack. The banana and almond butter provide natural sweetness, while the oats and cinnamon add texture and flavor. Enjoy!

How would you rate this dish?

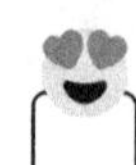 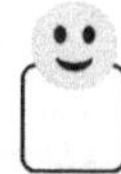 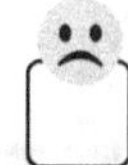 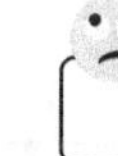 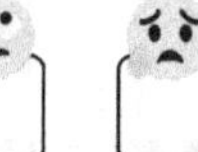

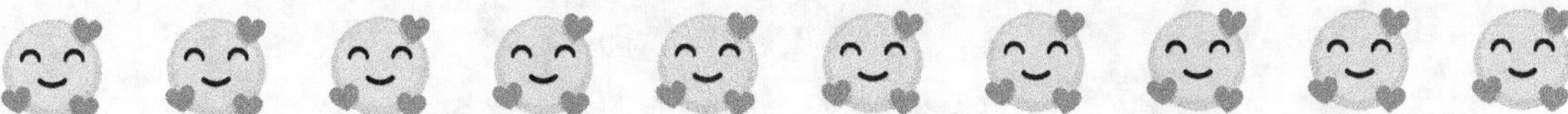

107. Whole-grain blueberry muffins

Prep Time :   Cook Time :    Servings :

Is this dish easy or difficult for you to make?

○   ○

Write 5 ....
friends
with   ....
whom
you   ....
want to
share   ....
this
dish   ....

INGREDIENTS

- 1 1/2 cups whole-wheat flour
- 1 cup rolled oats
- 1 teaspoon baking powder
- 1/2 teaspoon baking soda
- 1/4 teaspoon salt
- 1 cup plain Greek yogurt
- 1/2 cup honey
- 1 egg
- 1 teaspoon vanilla extract
- 1 cup fresh or frozen blueberries

1. Preheat the oven to 375°F. Grease a 12-cup muffin tin or line with paper liners.

2. In a medium bowl, whisk together the whole-wheat flour, rolled oats, baking powder, baking soda, and salt.

3. In a separate bowl, combine the Greek yogurt, honey, egg, and vanilla extract. Mix well.

4. Gently fold the wet ingredients into the dry ingredients just until combined. Fold in the blueberries.

5. Scoop the batter evenly into the prepared muffin cups, filling them about 3/4 full.

6. Bake for 18-20 minutes, until a toothpick inserted in the center comes out clean.

7. Allow the muffins to cool in the tin for 5 minutes before transferring to a wire rack to cool completely.

These whole-grain blueberry muffins are a great fertility-boosting snack for couples. The whole-wheat flour and oats provide complex carbohydrates, fiber, and B vitamins. Blueberries are rich in antioxidants, which can help support reproductive health. The Greek yogurt adds protein and probiotics. Enjoy these muffins as part of a balanced diet to help support fertility.

How would you rate this dish?

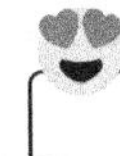 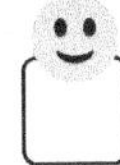  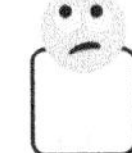 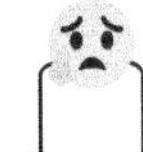

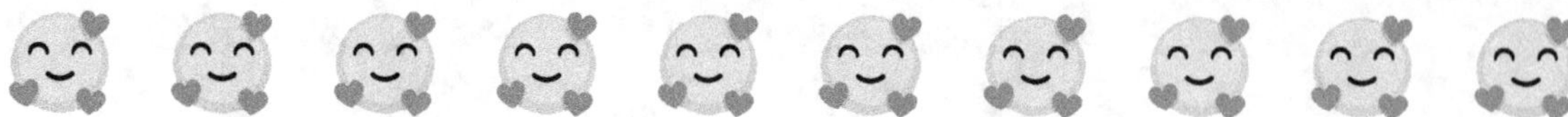

108. Greek yogurt with pomegranate seeds and honey

Let's do that and fill in the time here  Prep Time :   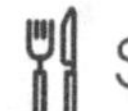 Cook Time :   Servings :

Is this dish easy or difficult for you to make?

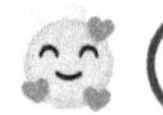 ◯   ◯

Write 5 friends with whom you want to share this dish

....

....

....

....

....

INGREDIENTS

- 1 cup plain Greek yogurt
- 1/2 cup pomegranate seeds
- 2 tablespoons honey

1. Scoop the Greek yogurt into a serving bowl or individual dish.

2. Sprinkle the pomegranate seeds over the top of the yogurt.

3. Drizzle the honey over the pomegranate seeds and yogurt.

That's it! This simple dish provides several fertility-boosting nutrients:

- Greek yogurt is high in protein, calcium, and probiotics, which are important for reproductive health.

- Pomegranate seeds are rich in antioxidants like vitamin C, folate, and polyphenols. These nutrients can help support egg and sperm quality.

- Honey contains natural sugars, vitamins, and minerals that may help regulate hormones and improve fertility.

This makes a delicious and nutritious breakfast, snack, or dessert for couples trying to conceive. The combination of protein, healthy fats, and antioxidants makes it a great fertility-supporting option.

Feel free to adjust the amounts of each ingredient to your taste. You can also add a sprinkle of cinnamon or chopped nuts for extra flavor and nutrients. Enjoy!

How would you rate this dish?

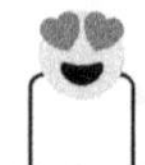 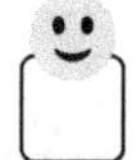  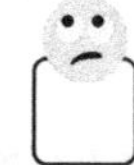 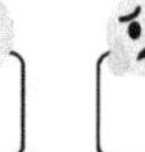 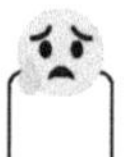

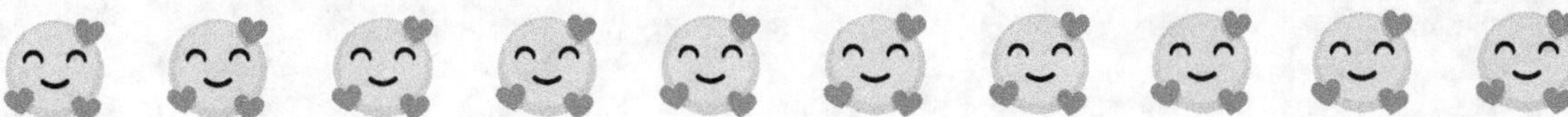

109. Homemade granola bars with nuts and dried fruit

Prep Time :   Cook Time :   Servings :

Is this dish easy or difficult for you to make?

 ◯   😊 ◯

Write 5 friends with whom you want to share this dish ....

INGREDIENTS

- 2 cups rolled oats
- 1/2 cup chopped nuts (such as almonds, walnuts, or pecans)
- 1/2 cup shredded unsweetened coconut
- 1/4 cup ground flaxseed
- 1/4 cup honey
- 1/4 cup nut butter (such as almond or peanut butter)
- 1/4 cup dried fruit (such as chopped apricots, cranberries, or raisins)
- 1/2 teaspoon cinnamon
- 1/4 teaspoon salt

How would you rate this dish?

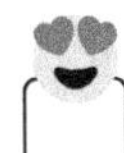 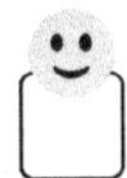 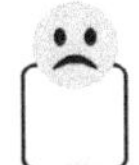 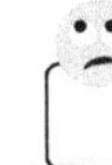 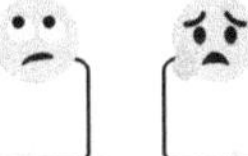

1. Preheat the oven to 325°F. Line an 8x8 inch baking pan with parchment paper, leaving some overhang on the sides.

2. In a large bowl, combine the rolled oats, chopped nuts, shredded coconut, and ground flaxseed. Mix well.

3. In a small saucepan, heat the honey and nut butter over low heat, stirring constantly, until smooth and combined.

4. Pour the honey-nut butter mixture over the dry ingredients and stir until everything is well coated.

5. Fold in the dried fruit, cinnamon, and salt.

6. Press the mixture firmly into the prepared baking pan, using your hands or the back of a spoon to compact it.

7. Bake for 20-25 minutes, until the edges are lightly golden.

8. Allow the granola bars to cool completely in the pan before lifting them out using the parchment paper overhang. Cut into bars or squares.

These homemade granola bars are packed with fertility-boosting nutrients:

- Oats, nuts, and seeds provide complex carbohydrates, protein, healthy fats, and fiber.
- Honey and dried fruit offer natural sweetness and antioxidants.
- The combination of ingredients can help support hormone balance, egg and sperm quality, and overall reproductive health.

Enjoy these bars as a nutritious snack or breakfast for couples trying to conceive.

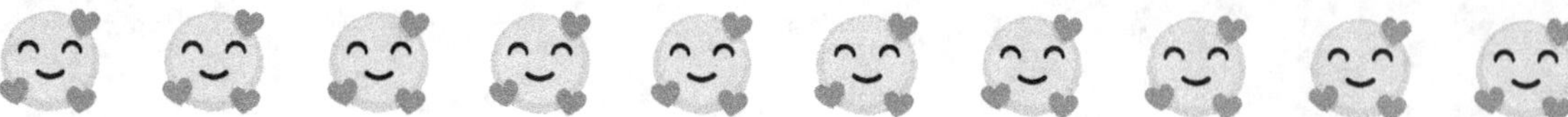

110. Baked pears with a sprinkle of cinnamon

Prep Time :   Cook Time :   Servings :

Is this dish easy or difficult for you to make?

 ◯   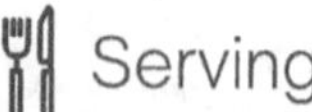 ◯

Write 5 ....
friends
with ....
whom
you ....
want to
share ....
this
dish ....

INGREDIENTS

- 4 ripe but firm pears, halved and cored
- 2 tablespoons unsalted butter, melted
- 2 tablespoons brown sugar
- 1 teaspoon ground cinnamon
- 1/4 teaspoon ground nutmeg (optional)

1. Preheat your oven to 375°F (190°C).

2. Arrange the pear halves, cut-side up, in a baking dish or on a rimmed baking sheet.

3. In a small bowl, mix together the melted butter, brown sugar, cinnamon, and nutmeg (if using).

4. Spoon the butter-sugar mixture evenly over the top of the pear halves, making sure to get some in the cavities where the cores were.

5. Bake for 20-25 minutes, or until the pears are tender when pierced with a fork. The tops should be lightly browned and caramelized.

6. Serve the baked pears warm, drizzling any extra juices from the baking dish over the top.

These baked pears make a wonderful, naturally sweet and comforting dessert or snack. The cinnamon and nutmeg add warmth and depth of flavor, complementing the juicy pears perfectly.

Pears are a great fruit choice for couples trying to conceive, as they are a good source of fiber, vitamins, and antioxidants that can support overall reproductive health. The cinnamon also has anti-inflammatory properties that may be beneficial.

Enjoy these baked pears on their own or with a dollop of Greek yogurt or a sprinkle of chopped nuts for added nutrition.

How would you rate this dish?

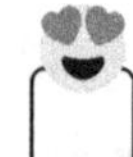 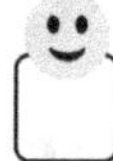  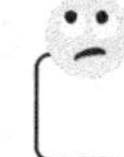 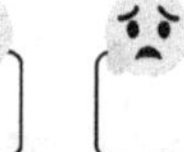

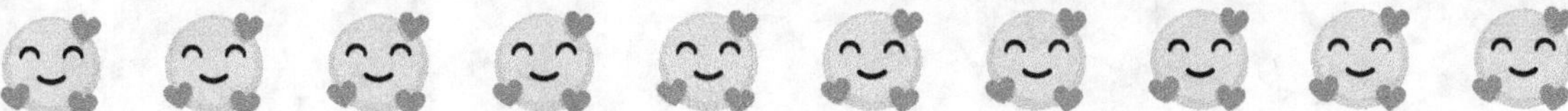

111. Green smoothie with kale, apple, and ginger

 Prep Time :   Cook Time :   Servings :

Is this dish easy or difficult for you to make?

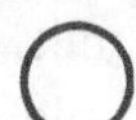 ◯    ◯

Write 5 friends with whom you want to share this dish ....

INGREDIENTS

- 1 cup packed kale leaves, stems removed
- 1 cup unsweetened almond milk (or milk of your choice)
- 1 medium apple, cored and chopped
- 1-inch piece of fresh ginger, peeled and grated
- 1 tablespoon ground flaxseed
- 1 tablespoon honey (optional)
- 1 cup ice cubes

1. Add the kale and almond milk to a high-speed blender. Blend on high speed until the kale is fully incorporated and the mixture is smooth.

2. Add the chopped apple, grated ginger, ground flaxseed, and honey (if using). Blend again until well combined and smooth.

3. Add the ice cubes and blend on high speed until the smoothie is thick and creamy.

4. Pour the green smoothie into a glass and enjoy immediately.

This green smoothie is packed with fertility-boosting nutrients:

- Kale is a nutrient-dense leafy green that's rich in vitamins A, C, and K, as well as folate and antioxidants.
- Apples provide fiber, vitamin C, and polyphenols that can help support reproductive health.
- Ginger has anti-inflammatory properties and may help regulate hormones.
- Flaxseed is a great source of omega-3 fatty acids, which are important for egg and sperm quality.

The combination of these ingredients creates a delicious and nourishing smoothie that can be a great addition to a fertility-friendly diet. Feel free to adjust the amounts of each ingredient to your taste.

Enjoy this green smoothie as a nutritious breakfast, snack, or anytime you need a boost of fertility-supporting nutrients.

How would you rate this dish?

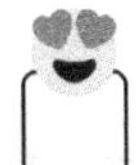 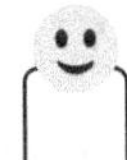  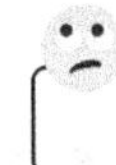 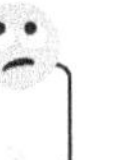

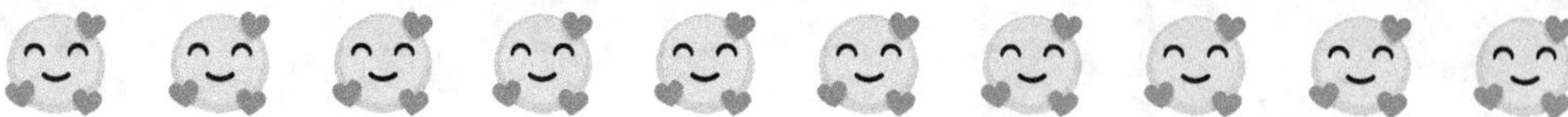

112. Berry and spinach smoothie with almond milk

Let's do that and fill in the time here

 Prep Time :　　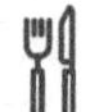 Cook Time :　　Servings :

Is this dish easy or difficult for you to make?

Write 5 friends with whom you want to share this dish

....
....
....
....
....

INGREDIENTS

- 1 cup fresh or frozen mixed berries (such as strawberries, blueberries, raspberries)
- 1 cup packed fresh spinach leaves
- 1 cup unsweetened almond milk
- 1 tablespoon ground flaxseed
- 1 tablespoon honey (optional)
- 1 cup ice cubes

1. Add the mixed berries, spinach, almond milk, ground flaxseed, and honey (if using) to a high-speed blender.

2. Blend on high speed until the mixture is smooth and creamy, about 1-2 minutes.

3. Add the ice cubes and blend again until the smoothie is thick and well-chilled.

4. Pour the smoothie into a glass and enjoy immediately.

This Berry and Spinach Smoothie is a nutrient-dense and fertility-supporting drink:

- Berries are rich in antioxidants, vitamins, and fiber, which can help support egg and sperm health.
- Spinach is a great source of folate, iron, and other important vitamins and minerals for reproductive health.
- Almond milk provides a dairy-free, calcium-rich base for the smoothie.
- Flaxseed is a good source of omega-3 fatty acids and lignans, which can help regulate hormones.
- Honey (if used) adds natural sweetness and contains antioxidants.

This smoothie makes a great breakfast, snack, or anytime treat for couples trying to conceive. The combination of berries, greens, and healthy fats provides a powerful boost of fertility-supporting nutrients.

Feel free to adjust the amounts of each ingredient to your taste preferences. You can also add other nutrient-dense ingredients like chia seeds, Greek yogurt, or a scoop of protein powder.

Enjoy this delicious and nourishing Berry and Spinach Smoothie!

How would you rate this dish?

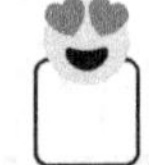 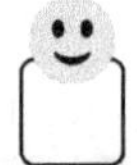  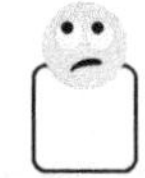 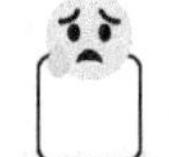

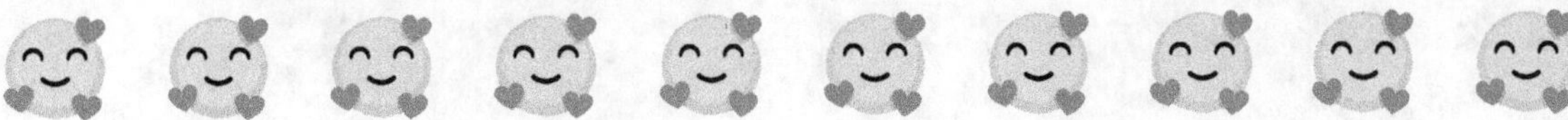

113. Freshly squeezed orange juice

 Prep Time :　　🕐 Cook Time :　　🍴 Servings :

Is this dish easy or difficult for you to make?

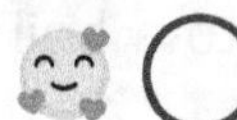 ◯　　　◯

Write 5 friends with whom you want to share this dish

....

....

....

....

INGREDIENTS

- 4-6 medium-sized oranges, washed

1. Roll the oranges on the counter with the palm of your hand to help release the juices.

2. Cut the oranges in half crosswise.

3. Using a citrus juicer or reamer, squeeze the juice from each orange half into a pitcher or container.

4. Stir the juice to combine all the different orange varieties.

5. Optionally, you can strain the juice through a fine-mesh sieve to remove any pulp or seeds.

6. Serve the freshly squeezed orange juice immediately, over ice if desired.

Tips:
- Use a variety of orange types (e.g. navel, Valencia, blood orange) for a more complex flavor.
- Refrigerate any leftover juice in an airtight container for up to 3-4 days.
- For a sweeter juice, you can add a touch of honey or agave nectar.

Freshly squeezed orange juice is a wonderful source of vitamin C, which is important for fertility and reproductive health. The antioxidants in orange juice may also help support egg and sperm quality.

Enjoy this refreshing and nutrient-dense juice as part of a balanced, fertility-friendly diet. It makes a great breakfast or snack for couples trying to conceive.

How would you rate this dish?

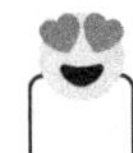 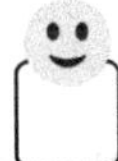  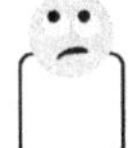 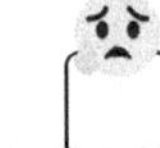

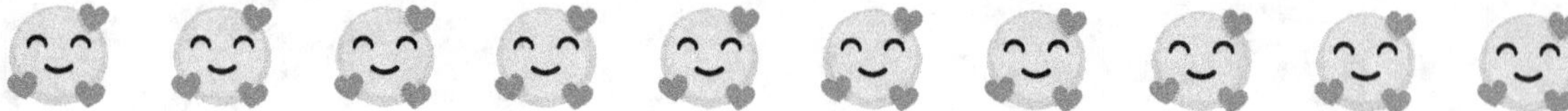

114. Herbal tea with lemon and honey

  Prep Time : 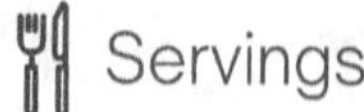 Cook Time : 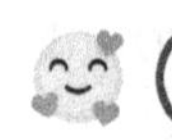 Servings :

Is this dish easy or difficult for you to make?

Write 5 friends with whom you want to share this dish

....

....

....

....

....

INGREDIENTS

- 1 cup boiling water
- 1 herbal tea bag (such as chamomile, ginger, or peppermint)
- 1 tablespoon freshly squeezed lemon juice
- 1-2 teaspoons honey (to taste)

1. Bring 1 cup of water to a boil in a small saucepan or kettle.

2. Place the herbal tea bag in a mug or teapot. Pour the boiling water over the tea bag.

3. Allow the tea to steep for 5-7 minutes, or according to the package instructions.

4. Remove the tea bag and stir in the freshly squeezed lemon juice.

5. Add 1-2 teaspoons of honey, to taste. Stir until the honey is fully dissolved.

6. Enjoy the tea warm, sipping slowly.

This herbal tea with lemon and honey can be a soothing and nourishing beverage for couples trying to conceive:

- Herbal teas like chamomile, ginger, and peppermint can help reduce stress and promote relaxation, which is important for fertility.
- Lemon provides a boost of vitamin C, an antioxidant that may help support egg and sperm health.
- Honey contains natural sugars, vitamins, and minerals that may help regulate hormones and improve fertility.

The combination of the warm, comforting tea with the bright, tangy lemon and sweet honey creates a delicious and fertility-friendly drink.

Feel free to experiment with different herbal tea varieties or add a cinnamon stick, a slice of fresh ginger, or a sprinkle of nutmeg for extra flavor and health benefits.

Enjoy this Herbal Tea with Lemon and Honey as a relaxing and nourishing beverage throughout the day.

How would you rate this dish?

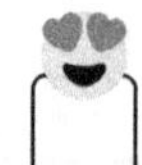 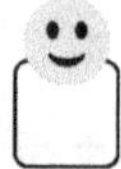  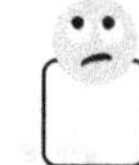 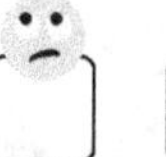

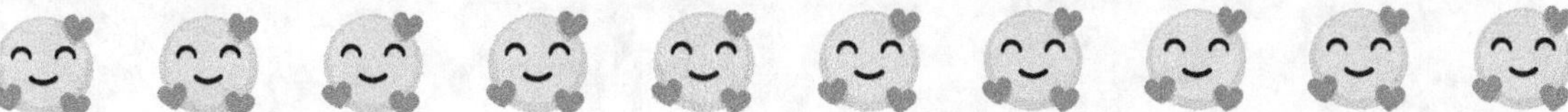

115. Matcha green tea with a splash of almond milk

 Prep Time :   Cook Time :   Servings :

Is this dish easy or difficult for you to make?

◯   ◯

Write 5 friends with whom you want to share this dish

....
....
....
....

INGREDIENTS

- 1 teaspoon high-quality matcha green tea powder
- 1 cup hot water (just below boiling)
- 2-3 tablespoons unsweetened almond milk
- Honey or maple syrup (optional)

1. In a small bowl or matcha whisk, add the matcha green tea powder.

2. Slowly pour in the hot water and whisk the mixture vigorously until it becomes frothy and smooth, with no lumps.

3. Pour the matcha tea into a mug.

4. Add 2-3 tablespoons of unsweetened almond milk, to taste. Stir gently to combine.

5. If desired, sweeten with a small drizzle of honey or maple syrup.

That's it! Your Matcha Green Tea with Almond Milk is ready to enjoy.

This drink is a great choice for couples trying to conceive due to the following benefits:

- Matcha is packed with antioxidants, L-theanine, and other nutrients that may help support fertility and reproductive health.
- Almond milk provides a dairy-free, calcium-rich base that is gentle on the digestive system.
- The combination of matcha and almond milk creates a creamy, soothing beverage that can help promote relaxation.

Feel free to adjust the amount of matcha powder and almond milk to your personal taste preferences. You can also experiment with adding a touch of cinnamon, vanilla, or a small amount of honey or maple syrup for extra flavor.

Enjoy this Matcha Green Tea with Almond Milk as a healthy, fertility-supporting beverage throughout the day.

How would you rate this dish?

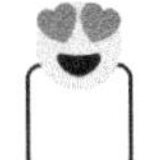 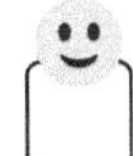 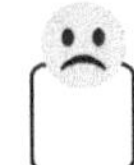 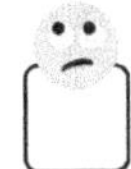 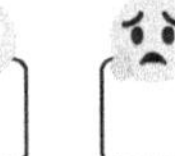

www.ingramcontent.com/pod-product-compliance
Lightning Source LLC
Chambersburg PA
CBHW081308250726

48662CB00008B/2452